Essential Best of Five and Multiple Choice Questions
for
Medical Finals
Third Edition

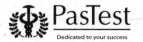

PasTest
Dedicated to your success

Essential Best of Five and Multiple Choice Questions
for
Medical Finals
Third Edition

Rema Kaur Wasan BA MBBS MA MRCP FRCR
Consultant Radiologist
King's College Hospital, London

Delilah Hassanally BSc MBBS MSc FRCS
Consultant Surgeon
Medway Hospital, Kent

Balvinder Singh Wasan BSc MBBS MRCP
Consultant Cardiologist
Queen Elizabeth Hospital, London

Ian Bickle MB MCh BAO(Hons)
Specialist Registrar Radiology
North Trent & Sheffield Training Scheme
Sheffield

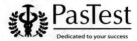

PasTest
Dedicated to your success

© 2006 PASTEST LTD
Egerton Court
Parkgate Estate
Knutsford
Cheshire
WA16 8DX

Telephone: 01565 752000

First published 1997
Second edition 2002
Third edition 2006

ISBN 1 904627 80 3
ISBN 978 1 904627 807

A catalogue record for this book is available from the British Library.

The information contained within this book was obtained by the authors from reliable sources. However, while every effort has been made to ensure its accuracy, no responsibility for loss, damage or injury occasioned to any person acting or refraining from action as a result of information contained herein can be accepted by the publishers or authors.

Typeset by Saxon Graphics Ltd, Derby
Printed and bound by Antony Rowe Ltd, Chippenham, Wiltshire

CONTENTS

ACKNOWLEDGEMENTS

Thanks to Dr Andy Bickle MBChB, BMedSc, MRCPsych, PGDip (Dist), Specialist Registrar in Forensic Psychiatry, East Midland centre for Forensic Mental Health for the contribution of the five psychiatric Best of Five MCQs.

INTRODUCTION

The aim of this book is to provide 'real' MCQ practice examinations at the appropriate level for undergraduates sitting their final medical examinations. These questions will also benefit those sitting the PLAB examination.

This book contains four test papers designed to be similar in format, content and balance of subjects to medical finals MCQ examinations. Answers and detailed teaching notes are given for each question. The questions are as 'real' as possible; they include material that has been remembered by medical students after their medical finals examinations. There is a natural tendency to recall the harder and more confusing topics, but rather than avoiding these, we have deliberately included them and so the pass mark for each paper is probably a little less than 50%. We hope medical students will use this to their advantage; everyone will get the easy questions right, but the medical student who enters the examination having done the more difficult questions should not just pass, but pass well.

We are delighted to include within the third edition a range of Best of Five MCQs. This is to reflect the change in the type of MCQs used in examinations at both undergraduate and postgraduate level. This addition has offered the opportunity to include new topics and questions related to contemporary practice. Extensive consultation with current students has taken place during the writing process to include relevant topics pitched at the right level to accommodate final year students' needs, with a fair balance of specialties covered. Furthermore comprehensive answers have been tailored to act as concise 'mini tutorials' on the themes covered.

Rema Wasan
Delilah Hassanally
Balvinder Wasan
Ian Bickle

MCQ EXAMINATION TECHNIQUE

Before sitting an MCQ examination, you will need to know how many questions are likely to be on the paper and how long you will be given to complete it. Thus you will be able to assess the approximate amount of time that can be spent on each question. Pacing yourself accurately during the examination to finish on time, or with time to spare, is essential.

In MCQ examinations you must read the question (both stem and items A–E) carefully. Take care not to mark the wrong boxes and think very carefully before making a mark on the answer sheet. There are two types of MCQs: True/False and Best of Five. Both are featured in each of the four exam papers in this book.

For True/False MCQ's regard each item as being independent of every other item – each refers to a specific quantum of knowledge. The item (or the stem and the item taken together) make up a statement for True/False MCQs. You are required to indicate whether you regard this statement as 'true' or 'false'. You must answer each stem. Look only at a single statement when answering – disregard all the other statements presented in the question. They have nothing to do with the item you are concentrating on.

The technique of approaching Best of Five MCQs is different. Remember that as the answer is the 'best of five' all five stems offered must be analyzed. Consider all the details in the stem – usually a clinical scenario. Look for clues. Fish out the red herrings. Try to think of the answer before viewing the stems. That way if your answer is included in the stems you will be a winner! More than one stem can be correct – it is the MOST correct which is right. One will frequently find it easy to narrow down the answers to two stems. The challenge is making the final correct decision.

Good luck from us all.

As you go through the questions, you can either mark your answers immediately on the answer sheet or you can mark them on the question paper and then transfer them to the answer sheet. If you adopt the second approach you must take great care not to make any errors and not to run out of time, since you will not be allowed extra time to transfer marks to the answer sheet. The answer sheet must always be marked neatly and carefully according to the instructions given. Careless marking is probably one of the commonest causes of rejection of answer sheets by the document reader.

- Do as many good quality practice papers as possible. This will help you to identify your strengths and weaknesses in time for further study. You can also use the Revision Index at the back of this book to find questions on specific topics, so that after you have done some reading you can test your knowledge.

- With the four exams provided in this book be strict with yourself and work under realistic exam conditions. You should develop an understanding of your own work rate so that you know how much time you can spend on each question.

- Read each question several times. Nobody at this vital stage in their career should be wasting marks because they misread or misunderstood the question.

- Each exam in this book contains 60 questions (15 Best of Five and 45 True/False Questions).

- If you have to guess the answer to a question, put a special mark next to it. You will then be able to find out if you are a good guesser. This is especially important if your examination is negatively marked, i.e. marks will be deducted for incorrect answers. It is important to know what you know as well as what you don't know.

- Use the Revision Checklist on the following pages to keep a record of the subjects you have covered and feel confident about. This will ensure that you do not miss out any key topics.

SAMPLE ANSWER SHEET

UNIVERSITY OF LONDON Management Systems Division

MULTIPLE-CHOICE EXAMINATION ANSWER SHEET

	Candidate No.	Test No.	College No.

DATE..................................

SURNAME..................................

FIRST NAME(S)..................................

Instructions: Use the HB pencil provided. To make an answer draw a single horizontal line along the dotted line above the appropriate letter or number. To answer 'TRUE' draw your line above the capital letter in the upper row. To answer 'FALSE' draw your line above the lower case letter in the lower row. For example:

[A] for 'TRUE'   [A] for 'FALSE'
[a]   [a]

If you change your mind and wish to cancel a completed answer, draw another line below the letter or number, along the dotted line. **Do not rub out.**

Candidate No. / Test No. / College No. number grids:
[0] [0] [0] [0]   [0] [0] [0] [0]   [0] [0]
[1] [1] [1] [1]   [1] [1] [1] [1]   [1] [1]
[2] [2] [2] [2]   [P] [2] [2] [2]   [2] [2]
[3] [3] [3] [3]   [3] [3] [3]   [3] [3]
[4] [4] [4] [4]   [4] [4] [4]   [4] [4]
[5] [5] [5] [5]   [5] [5] [5]   [5] [5]
[6] [6] [6] [6]   [6] [6] [6]   [6] [6]
[7] [7] [7] [7]   [7] [7] [7]   [7] [7]
[8] [8] [8] [8]   [8] [8] [8]   [8] [8]
[9] [9] [9] [9]   [9] [9] [9]   [9] [9]

Shown below is the correct method of completion, the correct method of cancellation/alteration and examples of various incorrect methods of completion.

CORRECT METHOD OF COMPLETION

True = [A]   False = [A]
       [a]   [a]

CORRECT METHOD OF CANCELLATION/ALTERATION

To cancel a response, draw a line below the letter. Do not rub out. Thus:

[A] or [A] = Cancelled
[a]   [a]

To alter a response, first cancel. Then draw a line above the other letter. Thus:

False = [A]   True = [A]
        [a]   [a]

INCORRECT METHODS OF COMPLETION

Too faint   [A]
Slanted   [A]
Too low   [A]
Too high   [A]
Into next box   [A] [B]
Too short   [A] [A] [A]
Isolated cancellation [A]
DETERMINATE TYPE T

Answer grid (numbered 1–66), each with rows:
[A] [B] [C] [D] [E]
[a] [b] [c] [d] [e]

Reproduced by kind permission of the University of London.

X

REVISION CHECKLIST

Use this checklist to record your revision progress. Tick the subjects when you feel confident that you have covered them adequately. This will ensure that you do not forget to revise any key topics. This list is arranged in approximate order of importance. Items closest to the top of each list are most likely to come up in examinations.

CARDIOLOGY
- ❏ Arrhythmias
- ❏ Atrial fibrillation
- ❏ Heart block
  - ❏ first degree, second degree
  - ❏ complete heart block
- ❏ Ventricular tachycardia
- ❏ Ventricular fibrillation
- ❏ Wolff-Parkinson-White syndrome
- ❏ Sick sinus syndrome
- ❏ Electrocardiogram (ECG) components and changes in: angina; pericarditis; myocardial infarction; hypothermia; common arrhythmias
- ❏ JVP waveform
- ❏ Cardiac failure
- ❏ Ischaemic heart disease
- ❏ Angina
- ❏ Myocardial infarction
- ❏ Pericardial disease
- ❏ Hypertension
  - ❏ primary
  - ❏ secondary
- ❏ Valvular dysfunction, in particular aortic, mitral. Some questions about Carey-Coombs, Austin Flint and Graham Steel murmurs have appeared in past papers
- ❏ Endocarditis
- ❏ Rheumatic fever
- ❏ Features of HOCM
- ❏ Marfan's syndrome

RESPIRATORY SYSTEM
- ❏ Bronchial carcinoma
- ❏ Asthma
- ❏ Pleural effusion
- ❏ COAD
- ❏ Pneumonia

- ❑ Cystic fibrosis
- ❑ Lung fibrosis
- ❑ Asbestos exposure
- ❑ Sarcoidosis
- ❑ Haemoptysis
- ❑ Tuberculosis

GASTROENTEROLOGY

- ❑ Peptic ulceration
- ❑ Dysphagia
- ❑ Jaundice
- ❑ Fat malabsorption
- ❑ Cirrhosis
- ❑ Hepatitis – drug or metabolic causes
- ❑ Crohn's disease
- ❑ Ulcerative colitis
- ❑ Hepatic encephalopathy
- ❑ Irritable bowel syndrome
- ❑ Diverticular disease
- ❑ Bowel malignancy
- ❑ Zollinger-Ellison syndrome – an uncommon condition but a common question in examinations
- ❑ Pernicious anaemia

NEUROPATHY

- ❑ Stroke
- ❑ Spastic paraparesis
- ❑ Multiple sclerosis
- ❑ Motor neurone disease
- ❑ Parkinson's disease
- ❑ Cerebellar lesion
- ❑ Frontal lobe syndrome
- ❑ Visual field defects
- ❑ Papilloedema
- ❑ Peripheral neuropathy
- ❑ Ptosis
- ❑ Reflexes
- ❑ Myasthenia gravis
- ❑ Meningitis
- ❑ Plantar responses
- ❑ Epilepsy – especially clinical features of TLE and management of status epilepticus
- ❑ Dementia
- ❑ Carpal tunnel syndrome

BEST OF FIVE AND MULTIPLE CHOICE QUESTIONS PAPER 1

60 questions: time allowed 2½ hours

Best of Five Questions
Mark your answers with a tick (True) in the box provided.

1.1   **A 53-year-old woman presents complaining of 'flashbacks'. Two months earlier she had been standing at a bus stop when a car swerved off the road into the queue, killing instantly a child standing near to her. Every day she experiences intrusive images of the child's face as it saw the car mount the curb. She has not been able to go to that part of town since the day and she has avoided taking the bus anywhere. She feels she is always on edge and jumps at the slightest noise around the house. She thinks things are getting worse rather than better and asks you whether there are any psychological treatments that might help her. Which one of the following approaches is indicated?**

- ❑   A   Psychodynamic therapy
- ❑   B   Cognitive behavioural therapy
- ❑   C   Supportive therapy
- ❑   D   Hypnotherapy
- ❑   E   Watchful waiting

1.2   **A 54-year-old 80-kg lady suffers an acute coronary syndrome (ACS) following an elective cholecystectomy. She was previously well and on no regular medications. ECG: T wave inversion in lateral leads. Troponin I (12-h sample): 0.26 µg/l. Which one of the following combination of drugs should be given immediately?**

- ❑   A   Aspirin 75 mg, clopidogrel 75 mg, enoxaparin 120 mg
- ❑   B   Aspirin 300 mg, enoxaparin 80 mg
- ❑   C   Clopidogrel 300 mg, enoxaparin 80 mg
- ❑   D   Aspirin 300 mg, clopidogrel 75 mg, enoxaparin 120 mg
- ❑   E   Aspirin 300 mg, clopidogrel 300 mg, enoxaparin 80 mg

1.3   A 32-year-old paediatric nurse complains of tiredness, generalised joint discomfort and a facial rash. She has recently returned from Portugal and states that the rash is worse. On examination: no active small joint synovitis; prominent erythematous facial rash. Blood tests reveal: haemoglobin 10.3 g/dl, MCV 88.8 fl, platelets 99×10⁹/l, WCC 2.8×10⁹/l. Which one of the following treatments is most appropriate at this stage?

- ❑   A   Methotrexate
- ❑   B   Sun avoidance
- ❑   C   Infliximab
- ❑   D   Hydroxychloroquine
- ❑   E   Azathioprine

1.4   A 68-year-old gentleman is admitted following a fall with a painful right knee. He has a history of osteoarthritis and atrial fibrillation (AF). Prior to admission he was independent and living alone. Whilst in casualty he gives a history of falling on his knee. Casualty staff reported an incident of urinary incontinence whilst in their care. No seizure activity was reported. Whilst on the ward he becomes sleepy, but rousable. Later in the night the nurses state he is no longer opening his eyes to voices and is making incomprehensible noises. What is the potential diagnosis which requires exclusion?

- ❑   A   Stroke
- ❑   B   A post ictal state
- ❑   C   Obstructive sleep apnoea
- ❑   D   Hypoglycaemia
- ❑   E   Subdural haematoma

1.5   A 32-year-old teacher is diagnosed with syringomyelia by her neurologist. She has sustained a number of burns to the hands unknowingly whilst cooking. Which one of the following combinations best fits the two sensory modalities carried in the damaged tract?

- ❑   A   Pain and dorsal tracts
- ❑   B   Pain and spinothalamic tract
- ❑   C   Proprioception and spinothalamic tract
- ❑   D   Fine touch and spinothalamic tract
- ❑   E   Proprioception and dorsal tracts

1.6   A 42-year-old lady attends a priority neurological outpatients clinic with a short but progressive history of double vision. It is noted by her husband that her speech would be worse last thing in the evening. She is a non-smoker and drinks 18 units a week of alcohol. Which one of the following is the best diagnostic test?

- ❏ A   Autoantibody to voltage-gated calcium channels
- ❏ B   Visually evoked responses
- ❏ C   CT brain
- ❏ D   CT chest
- ❏ E   Nerve conduction studies + repetitive nerve stimulation

1.7   A 41-year-old West Indian diplomat whilst on secondment in the UK develops an uncomfortable raised rash on the anterior aspects of both her lower legs. She has prided herself with her remarkably good health over the years despite recent visits with her work to Nigeria, Guyana and Vietnam. Which one of the following would be the best initial investigation to perform?

- ❏ A   Blood film
- ❏ B   Chest X-ray
- ❏ C   Ultrasound of the abdomen
- ❏ D   Stool microbiology
- ❏ E   Skin biopsy

1.8   An 18-year-old apprentice is referred by his GP with a query of bacterial meningitis. CT brain was normal. The patient complains of ongoing headache, photophobia and fever. Lumbar puncture (LP) is to be performed. Which one of the following issues is most correct with regard to performing a lumbar puncture?

- ❏ A   Verbal consent for the procedure is sufficient
- ❏ B   Without exception is performed in the left lateral position
- ❏ C   Normal CSF opening pressure ranges 14–24 mmH$_2$O
- ❏ D   Should only take place following neuro-imaging
- ❏ E   A concurrent plasma glucose sample should be taken

1.9   Whilst acting as a medical volunteer for the St John's Ambulance at a local fete a 19-year-old man is brought to you with a swollen face and lips, accompanied by wheeze following a bee sting. He is finding it difficult to breath and his BP is 83/45 mmHg from a manual reading. What should be done next?

- A Give 1:1000 IV adrenaline + IV hydrocortisone
- B Observe and arrange transfer to casualty
- C Give IV hydrocortisone
- D Give 1:1000 IM adrenaline + IV hydrocortisone
- E Give 1:10,000 IV adrenaline + IV hydrocortisone

1.10 A 72-year-old retired electrician complains of increasing shortness of breath, weight loss and two episodes of haemoptysis over the past week. He is an ex-smoker of 40 pack years. On examination: stony dull right base, no breath sounds heard, decreased vocal resonance. Which one of the following statements regarding mesothelioma is most correct?

- A It is caused by asbestos and smoking
- B It has a 5-year survival of 15%
- C It is usually diagnosed by open biopsy
- D It may have a lag period of up to 50 years between exposure and diagnosis
- E It will cause a transudate pleural effusion

1.11 A 46-year-old nurse takes an overdose of paracetamol. A suicide note was left. Her only past health problem is long-standing, well-controlled epilepsy for which she takes carbamazepine. She is believed to have taken approximately 30 tablets. When she reached hospital, blood samples were taken. From a collateral history this is 6 h after ingestion. Blood investigations: Hb 14.1 g/dl, WCC 6.4 × 10^9/l, Plt 321 × 10^9/l, Na 134 mmol/l, K 3.6 mmol/l, urea 4.6 mmol/l, Cr 76 μmol/l, Bil 12 μmol/l, AST 45 iu/l, ALT 86 iu/l, GGT 74 iu/l, ALP 53 iu/l. Paracetamol level 110 mg/l. Which one of the following is the ideal treatment for this patient?

- A IV saline + 4-hourly LFTs and prothrombin time
- B Give activated charcoal and repeat LFTs after 4 h
- C Repeat paracetamol levels at 8 h post ingestion before deciding on treatment
- D Give oral methionine
- E Give IV *N*-acetylcysteine

1.12 You are asked to see a patient in the obstetric ward who is suffering from severe eclampsia. Two hours previously she began to bleed profusely from her cannula site. After checking her coagulation screen both her prothrombin time (PTT) and activated partial thromboplastin time (APTT) were elevated. Her D-dimer was markedly raised. Her platelets were only 16 × 10⁹/l, having been 198 × 10⁹/l yesterday. You are suspicious she has developed disseminated intravascular coagulation (DIC). Which one of the following tests would best confirm this?

- ❑ A Citrated platelets
- ❑ B Fibrinogen
- ❑ C Anti-thrombin III
- ❑ D Blood film
- ❑ E Von Willebrand factor

1.13 A 72-year-old lady with metastatic carcinoma of the breast is admitted to your ward, as her family are finding it difficult to cope with her deterioration over the past 2 weeks. She appears drowsy and lethargic. She has known hepatic and bony secondary lesions. Her admission blood tests are: Na 137 mmol/l, K 3.9 mmol/l, urea 7.9 mmol/l, Cr 98 μmol/l, Ca 3.13 mmol/l, PO₄³⁻ 0.87 mmol/l, Mg 0.91 mmol/l, Alb 37 g/l, Hb 10.3 g/dl, MCV 98.3 fl, WCC 8.1 × 10⁹/l, Plt 186 × 10⁹/l. What is the correct initial treatment for this lady's hypercalcaemia?

- ❑ A An IVI of pamidronate
- ❑ B No intervention
- ❑ C 3000 ml IV saline
- ❑ D Radiotherapy to her bony lesions
- ❑ E Oral prednisolone

1.14 A 44-year-old alcoholic is admitted following a fall. He has a large laceration on the side of his head and a collateral history is given by a passer-by to the paramedics. He is opening his eyes when asked to by the nurses. He responds to questioning but only with words that cannot be made out. When pressure is applied to his nailbed his arm is withdrawn. Which one of the following is the correct Glasgow Coma Scale assessment?

❏   A   E3V3M4
❏   B   E2V3M4
❏   C   E3V3M3
❏   D   E2V2M4
❏   E   E2V2M5

1.15   **A 27-year-old man asks to see you because he doesn't feel his normal self. Things haven't been right following his divorce 6 months ago. Over the last 4 weeks he has felt low for most of each day, especially in the mornings when he wakes up early. He has lost all interest in his usual activities. He has not been to any matches at the football club where he is a season ticket holder. It has occurred to him a couple of times that he would be better off just swallowing a bottle of tablets and getting away from it all, but he doesn't think he'd do it because his parents have been there supporting him when he needed it. There is no significant medical history or previous psychiatric history. Which one of the following treatments would be most suitable?**

❏   A   Fluoxetine
❏   B   Imipramine
❏   C   Lithium
❏   D   Electroconvulsive therapy
❏   E   Phenelzine

Multiple Choice Questions

Mark your answers with a tick (True) or a cross (False) in the box provided. Leave the box blank for 'Don't know'. Do not look at the answers until you have completed the whole question paper.

1.16 The following statements about peptic ulceration are true

- ❑ A Duodenal ulcers do not become malignant
- ❑ B Duodenal ulcers are more common than gastric ulcers
- ❑ C Gastric ulceration usually occurs with a normal or low acid production
- ❑ D Gastric ulcers are associated with blood group A
- ❑ E Spicy food may play a role in the aetiology

1.17 Causes of erythema nodosum include

- ❑ A Streptococcal sore throat
- ❑ B Sarcoid
- ❑ C Sulphonamides
- ❑ D Tuberculosis
- ❑ E Trauma

1.18 The following may be detected by urine dipstick

- ❑ A Microalbuminuria
- ❑ B Red cell casts
- ❑ C Bence–Jones proteins
- ❑ D White blood cells
- ❑ E Nitrite

1.19 The following are possible causes of a goitre

- ❑ A Pregnancy
- ❑ B Puberty
- ❑ C Graves' disease
- ❑ D Carbimazole
- ❑ E Exogenous iodine

1.20   Syncope is a recognised feature of

❑ A   Pertussis
❑ B   Ménière's disease
❑ C   Hypertrophic obstructive cardiomyopathy
❑ D   Complete heart block
❑ E   Paroxysmal tachycardia

1.21   Glycosuria may be found in

❑ A   Normal patients
❑ B   Cushing's syndrome
❑ C   Addison's disease
❑ D   Fanconi syndrome
❑ E   Acromegaly

1.22   Recognised causes of diarrhoea include

❑ A   Chronic pancreatitis
❑ B   Thyrotoxicosis
❑ C   Carcinoid syndrome
❑ D   Hyperparathyroidism
❑ E   Diabetes mellitus

1.23   Hypercalcaemia can occur in

❑ A   Pseudohypoparathyroidism
❑ B   Pseudopseudohypoparathyroidism
❑ C   Sarcoid
❑ D   Acute pancreatitis
❑ E   Paget's disease

1.24   The following statements about the normal chest X-ray are correct

❑ A   The left hemidiaphragm is lower than the right
❑ B   The left hilum is higher than the right
❑ C   The trachea is slightly to the left of the midline
❑ D   The heart appears larger on a PA film
❑ E   The horizontal fissure is normally visible on the left

1.25 Causes of papilloedema include

- ❑ A Hyperparathyroidism
- ❑ B Type II respiratory failure
- ❑ C Hypertension
- ❑ D Benign intracranial hypertension
- ❑ E Parasagittal meningioma

1.26 Cystic fibrosis

- ❑ A Occurs in 1 in 20,000 live births
- ❑ B Has sex-linked recessive inheritance
- ❑ C Causes clubbing
- ❑ D Usually leads to death in the early teens
- ❑ E Causes steatorrhoea

1.27 Pulmonary embolism often produces the following

- ❑ A Pleuritic chest pain
- ❑ B Tachypnoea, tachycardia and hypoxia
- ❑ C Loud P2
- ❑ D ECG pattern of S1 Q3 T3
- ❑ E Cardiomegaly

1.28 Dysphagia occurs with

- ❑ A Iron deficiency
- ❑ B Myasthenia gravis
- ❑ C Chagas disease
- ❑ D Anxiety
- ❑ E Pyloric stenosis

1.29 Acromegaly causes

- ❑ A Glycosuria
- ❑ B Blindness
- ❑ C Hypertension
- ❑ D Cardiomyopathy
- ❑ E Hepatomegaly

1.30   The risk of osteoporosis is increased in

❑   A   Asians
❑   B   Thyrotoxicosis
❑   C   Premature menopause
❑   D   Steroid therapy
❑   E   Heparin treatment

1.31   Ocular complications of diabetes mellitus include

❑   A   Retinitis pigmentosa
❑   B   Optic neuritis
❑   C   New vessel formation in the retina
❑   D   An isolated third nerve palsy
❑   E   Glaucoma

1.32   The usual biochemical features of primary hyperaldosteronism include

❑   A   Hypokalaemia
❑   B   Hypernatraemia
❑   C   Metabolic acidosis
❑   D   Increased plasma renin activity
❑   E   Hypotension

1.33   The following statements about type I (insulin-dependent) diabetes are true

❑   A   Diabetic nephropathy affects about 4% of all subjects
❑   B   Retinopathy is less common than with type II diabetes
❑   C   There is an increased frequency of HLA DR3
❑   D   Nephropathy is more common than retinopathy
❑   E   Insulin dosage must be decreased when illness prevents eating and drinking

1.34   Nephrotic syndrome may be caused by

❑   A   Congenital defects
❑   B   Systemic lupus erythematosus (SLE)
❑   C   Retinal vein thrombosis
❑   D   Interstitial nephritis
❑   E   Gold

1.35   In Paget's disease

❏   A   Symptoms are proportional to the degree of skeletal involvement
❏   B   Serum calcium is usually elevated
❏   C   Plasma acid phosphatase is elevated
❏   D   Cardiac failure is a recognised complication
❏   E   About 10% of patients develop osteosarcoma

1.36   The following enable a diagnosis of diabetes mellitus to be made

❏   A   Random plasma glucose of 12 mmol/l
❏   B   Fasting plasma glucose of 6.8 mmol/l
❏   C   Islet cell antibodies
❏   D   Glycosuria
❏   E   Retinal new vessel formation

1.37   The following are causes of a ptosis

❏   A   Dystrophia myotonica
❏   B   Myasthenia gravis
❏   C   Facial nerve palsy
❏   D   Damage to the parasympathetic nervous system
❏   E   Damage to the sympathetic nervous system

1.38   The following may be features of a Bell's palsy

❏   A   Pain
❏   B   Hyperacusis
❏   C   Loss of taste in the anterior part of the tongue
❏   D   Ptosis
❏   E   Deafness

1.39   The following may be presenting features of acute myocardial infarction

❏   A   Confusion
❏   B   Acute pulmonary oedema
❏   C   Syncope
❏   D   Diabetic hyperglycaemic states
❏   E   Fall

1.40   Cardiac causes of finger clubbing include

❑ A   Transposition of the vessels
❑ B   Maladie de Roger
❑ C   Atrial septal defect
❑ D   Rheumatic fever
❑ E   Fallot's tetralogy

1.41   In the management of a cardiac arrest

❑ A   DC cardioversion is seldom useful in ventricular fibrillation
❑ B   External cardiac compression should depress the sternum 4–5 cm (1.5–2 in)
❑ C   Hypovolaemia may be a cause of electromechanical dissociation
❑ D   Sodium bicarbonate must be given to prevent acidosis
❑ E   Calcium chloride is recommended for asystole

1.42   The following diseases and antibodies are associated

	Antibody	*Disease*
❑ A	Antimitochondrial	CREST
❑ B	Rheumatoid factor	Rheumatoid arthritis
❑ C	Anti-double-stranded DNA	SLE
❑ D	Anticardiolipin	SLE
❑ E	Anti-centromere	Primary biliary cirrhosis

1.43   The following apply to the management of chronic obstructive pulmonary disease (COPD)

❑ A   In the treatment of an exacerbation, 24% oxygen should be used initially
❑ B   Long-term oxygen has been shown to improve life expectancy
❑ C   Influenza vaccine is contraindicated
❑ D   In an infective exacerbation the most likely organism is *Staphylococcus aureus*
❑ E   Regular blood transfusions may help to increase oxygen-carrying capacity

1.44   Spontaneous rib fracture may be caused by

❏ A   Coughing
❏ B   Metastases
❏ C   Primary lung tumour
❏ D   Pneumothorax
❏ E   Osteoporosis

1.45   Rapid respiration may be caused by

❏ A   Hyperosmolar ketoacidosis
❏ B   Salicylate overdose
❏ C   Hypoglycaemia
❏ D   Lesions of the pons
❏ E   Anxiety

1.46   The following are causes of a pleural effusion

❏ A   Pancreatitis
❏ B   Ovarian carcinoma
❏ C   Retroperitoneal fibrosis
❏ D   Mesothelioma
❏ E   Pulmonary infarction

1.47   The following are associated with dilatation of the pupil

❏ A   Complete third nerve palsy
❏ B   Horner's syndrome
❏ C   Entering the garden on a bright day
❏ D   Old age
❏ E   Convergence

1.48   Spontaneous pneumothorax

❏ A   Usually occurs in men
❏ B   Is best treated with positive pressure ventilation
❏ C   May be managed by observation alone
❏ D   If left alone, a 100% pneumothorax would take 2–3 weeks to fully re-expand
❏ E   Is often caused by rib fractures

1.49   Recognised features of sarcoidosis include

☐ A   Lymphocytosis
☐ B   Lupus pernio
☐ C   Facial nerve palsy
☐ D   Splenomegaly
☐ E   Bilateral hilar lymphadenopathy

1.50   The following can be attributed to a urinary tract infection in an elderly person

☐ A   Falls
☐ B   Disorientation
☐ C   Urinary incontinence
☐ D   Anaemia
☐ E   Wandering at night

1.51   Portosystemic encephalopathy may be precipitated by

☐ A   Gastrointestinal haemorrhage
☐ B   Lactulose
☐ C   Benzodiazepines
☐ D   Diuretics
☐ E   Constipation

1.52   The following apply to the arterial blood pressure

☐ A   On standing the systolic and diastolic pressures rise
☐ B   It increases on exercise
☐ C   There is a diurnal variation
☐ D   There may be a difference between the right and left brachial pressures
☐ E   It is falsely high when a small cuff is used

1.53   Causes of a collapsing pulse include

☐ A   Aortic regurgitation
☐ B   Thyrotoxicosis
☐ C   Mitral stenosis
☐ D   Bradycardia
☐ E   Fever

1.54   The following statements on mortality rates are true

❏   A   The maternal mortality rate is the number of deaths of mothers attributable to pregnancy and delivery divided by the number of births

❏   B   The perinatal mortality rate is the number of deaths in the first week of life (excluding stillbirths) divided by the total number of births

❏   C   The neonatal mortality rate is the number of deaths in the first four weeks of life divided by the number of deaths in the first year

❏   D   The stillbirth rate is the number of babies born dead after 28 weeks divided by the number of live births

❏   E   The infant mortality rate is the number of deaths in the first year divided by the number of live births

1.55   The following apply to infectious diseases

❏   A   Since 1992 there has been a reduction in the incidence of *Haemophilus influenzae* type B infections in children

❏   B   There have been no confirmed cases of measles since 1994

❏   C   Smallpox was declared to have been eradicated from the world in the 1960s

❏   D   *H. influenzae* type B viruses are subject to antigenic shift

❏   E   Approximately 90% of adults are immune to the chickenpox virus

1.56   Immunisation is the main factor responsible for the reduction in rates of

❏   A   Pulmonary tuberculosis
❏   B   Diphtheria
❏   C   Whooping cough
❏   D   Cholera
❏   E   Measles

1.57   The following are side-effects of inhaled steroids

❏   A   Cataracts
❏   B   Oral candidiasis
❏   C   Hoarse voice
❏   D   Cushing's disease
❏   E   Adrenal suppression

1.58   Polyuria may result from

❑   A   Hypokalaemia
❑   B   Hypercalcaemia
❑   C   An epileptic attack
❑   D   Diabetes insipidus
❑   E   Hypoglycaemia

1.59   The following statements about systolic murmurs are true

❑   A   Mitral valve prolapse produces a pansystolic murmur
❑   B   The murmur of a ventricular septal defect is pansystolic
❑   C   Hypertrophic obstructive cardiomyopathy produces a murmur loudest on squatting
❑   D   An atrial septal defect produces an ejection systolic murmur
❑   E   Aortic stenosis produces an early systolic murmur

1.60   Leucocytes in the urine occur with

❑   A   Aspirin nephropathy
❑   B   Nephroblastoma
❑   C   Renal tuberculosis
❑   D   Retroperitoneal fibrosis
❑   E   Polycystic renal disease

———————————— **END** ————————————

**Go over your answers until your time is up. Correct answers
and teaching notes are overleaf**

BEST OF FIVE AND MULTIPLE CHOICE QUESTIONS PAPER 1
Answers

The correct answer options for each question are given below.

1.1	B		1.31	C D E
1.2	E		1.32	A B
1.3	D		1.33	C
1.4	E		1.34	A B E
1.5	B		1.35	D
1.6	E		1.36	A
1.7	B		1.37	A B E
1.8	E		1.38	A B C
1.9	D		1.39	A B C D E
1.10	D		1.40	A E
1.11	E		1.41	B C
1.12	D		1.42	B C D
1.13	C		1.43	A B
1.14	A		1.44	A B C E
1.15	A		1.45	A B D E
1.16	A B C		1.46	A B D E
1.17	A B C D		1.47	A
1.18	D E		1.48	A C
1.19	A B C D		1.49	A B C D E
1.20	A C D E		1.50	A B C
1.21	A B D E		1.51	A C D E
1.22	A B C E		1.52	B C D E
1.23	C E		1.53	A B E
1.24	A B		1.54	A E
1.25	B C D E		1.55	A B E
1.26	C E		1.56	B C E
1.27	A B		1.57	B C E
1.28	A B C D		1.58	A B D
1.29	A C D E		1.59	B C D
1.30	A B C D E		1.60	A B C

BEST OF FIVE AND MULTIPLE CHOICE QUESTIONS PAPER 1
Answers and Teaching Notes

1.1 B: Cognitive behavioural therapy

This woman has post traumatic stress disorder. This is a delayed and/or protracted response to a stressful event or situation of an exceptional nature which is likely to cause distress in almost anyone. Typical symptoms include repeated reliving of the trauma in intrusive 'flashbacks', vivid memories or dreams, avoidance of activities and situations reminiscent of the trauma, emotional numbness, detachment from other people and unresponsiveness to surroundings. There is usually autonomic arousal with a state of hypervigilance, an enhanced startle reaction and insomnia. Other depressive and anxiety symptoms may be seen.

Cognitive behavioural therapy (CBT) which focuses on the trauma and responses to the trauma is recommended by the National Institute for Clinical Excellence (NICE) in the UK. There is no convincing evidence of a clinically important effect for any of the other therapies. 'Watchful waiting' to see what happens is a valid approach if the symptoms are mild and have been present for less than 1 month after the trauma.

1.2 E: Aspirin 300 mg, clopidogrel 300 mg, enoxaparin 80 mg

Acute coronary syndrome (ACS) spans the spectrum of unstable angina and myocardial infarction. A troponin rise of 0.26 µgl/l in a previously healthy patient with no confounding factors such as renal impairment, accompanied by ischaemic ECG changes, represents a non ST elevation myocardial infarction (NSTEMI). Lysis is not indicated in this situation, but immediate treatment with antiplatelet agents and anticoagulation is essential. Analgesia, oxygen and nitrates would also be administered. When clinically appropriate an ACE inhibitor, statin and beta-blocker may be introduced. At diagnosis of the ischaemic event 300 mg of aspirin should be administered and the CURE trial (Clopidogrel in unstable angina to prevent recurrent events) has proven the value in giving the same dose of clopidogrel as a stat dose.

Additionally, low-molecular-weight heparin (LMWH; in the form of enoxaparin) is given as a 1 mg/kg twice daily dose.

The treatment dose of LMWH for pulmonary embolus is 1.5 mg/kg once daily (in this patient 120 mg). Aspirin and clopidogrel are both continued after the first dose at 75 mg once daily.

1.3 D: Hydroxychloroquine

This is a typical history of a patient with systemic lupus erythematosus (SLE). The challenge in this question lies in knowing how to treat appropriately given the clinical features. This question exemplifies the different approach the examiner may take in Best of Five MCQs. Either the diagnosis is straightforward from the information given and a specific question related to the disease is asked, or the information presented is more challenging but for the well read the diagnosis is clear.

Furthermore, SLE is one of a legion of systemic diseases, often with non-specific symptomatology, which can present itself in a host of clinical scenarios. Several of the treatments are suitable for managing SLE, the key lies in establishing which meets the patient's needs most correctly ('the best').

SLE sufferers with disease limited to the joints and skin will typically be tried first on hydroxychloroquine. This is an anti-malarial which has been found to be beneficial for those with disease limited to these organ systems. It is essential that patients on hydroxychloroquine are enrolled in some form of ophthalmology surveillance programme due to the small risks of developing drug-induced retinopathy. Disease-modifying anti-rheumatic drugs (DMARDS) are reserved for the treatment of more aggressive disease.

1.4 E: Subdural haematoma

Acute subdural haematoma is a life-threatening neurosurgical emergency. It is reversible if speedily diagnosed and acted upon. It is more common in the elderly and those on anticoagulant medications. A fluctuating conscious level in an elderly patient should always arouse suspicion.

From the history one should have extracted the vital clues

History of AF – may be on warfarin
Fall
Episode of urinary incontinence
Rapid drop in conscious level (GCS)/fluctuant GCS

All of the listed diagnoses may give a similar presentation, but the most important requiring prompt exclusion (even in the middle of the night) is a subdural haematoma. Urgent CT brain imaging would be indicated.

1.5 B: Pain and spinothalamic tract

Syringobulbia and syringomyelia are rare neurological conditions which are beautifully demonstrated by magnetic resonance imaging (MRI). A syrinx is an abnormal fluid-filled cavity which occurs in either the spinal cord (myelia) or the brainstem (bulbia). The syrinx contains cerebrospinal fluid (CSF). It is the pressure effects, often following expansion of the cavity over several years, that lead to neurological symptoms, and typically presentation is in the third and fourth decades of life. Involvement of the spinothalamic tracts which carry pain and temperature neurones leads to presentation with painless burns. Proprioception, fine touch, vibration and two-point discrimination are carried within the dorsal (posterior) columns.

1.6 E: Nerve conduction studies + repetitive nerve stimulation

Myasthenia gravis (MG) is an idiopathic disease in which antibodies develop against the acetylcholine receptor protein on the post synaptic membrane of a neurone. This interferes with the function of neurotransmission, presenting in the patient as weakness and fatigability. This fatigability is a cardinal feature of the disease with symptoms typically being worse in the evening or towards the end of a prolonged activity requiring the same muscles. For example weakness and fatigue of the ocular muscles after watching a lengthy evening TV programme.

Myasthenia gravis is associated in a considerable proportion of patients (especially the <40 year-old age group) with thymic hyperplasia or thymic tumours. For this reason CT chest imaging is indicated at the time of diagnosis. In the older patient diagnostic confusion may occur with the rare, but well documented, Eaton–Lambert myasthenic syndrome (LEMS). Clinically the difference is noted in testing muscle strength. In MG the muscle group repetitively tested will fatigue with time whereas the opposite occurs in LEMS. This can be objectively documented neurophysiologically by performing nerve conduction studies with repetitive nerve stimulation. Following the repeat stimulation of a nerve a decrement in the evoked muscle action is observed. Diagnosis may be further confirmed by the edrophonium (TENSILON) test.

1.7 B: Chest X-ray

This patient has erythema nodosum. It is more common in blacks than in Caucasians. Her extensive travel history may be contributory, although the commonest cause for this condition is idiopathic. One can be easily distracted in a question including foreign countries into assuming that a weird and wonderful infectious disease is responsible. It is not uncommon for examiners to include information that are 'red herrings' in order to distinguish the excellent candidates confident of their knowledge and its application from the rest of the field. Likewise it is tempting to go for the most direct investigation, in this case skin biopsy, without careful attention to the wording of the question. Skin biopsy may be the *best investigation* to ascertain a diagnosis but the *best initial investigation* is getting a chest X-ray (CXR). It is quick and excludes the most important potential causes of erythema nodosum: tuberculosis and sarcoidosis. Several stems may even be correct for the specific question but it is the best that counts – 'the best of five'.

1.8 E: A concurrent plasma glucose should be taken

Lumbar puncture (LP) may be a ward procedure but it is both invasive and not without complication. Written consent should be ascertained from the patient – providing they are of the right mind to comprehend the information and make a rational decision. Although routinely performed in the left lateral position it may be performed in the sitting position and is frequently the only way to successfully acquire cerebrospinal fluid (CSF) in the larger patient. Neuro-imaging is required before LP only in those patients in whom there is a clinical suspicion of raised intracranial pressure. LP *should not* be performed in those with an acutely raised CSF pressure as 'coning' of the brainstem may occur.

The normal range for opening pressure is 50–180 mmH$_2$O. In a patient with a clinical suspicion of bacterial meningitis plasma glucose is essential so the CSF: plasma glucose ratio can be calculated. A reduced ratio is a key distinguishing feature of bacterial meningitis, indicating the presence of bacteria within the CSF consuming glucose. The normal ratio is >2/3.

1.9 D: Give 1:1000 IM adrenaline + IV hydrocortisone

Anaphylaxis requires immediate treatment. Those with known anaphylactic reactions (often to a specific substance such as peanuts) carry their own treatment in the form of a preloaded syringe of adrenaline. When the symptoms are mild and vital signs are within normal range the administration of IV hydrocortisone and chlorpheniramine is sufficient with adrenaline available should symptoms become more profound. If circulatory failure develops (SHOCK) adrenaline should be administered. This takes the form of 1:1000 adrenaline by the intramuscular (IM) route. Note this is different to during cardiac arrest when it is 1:10,000 via an intravenous (IV) route. Hydrocortisone, even by an intravenous route, takes several hours to have an effect. It is the inotropic action of adrenaline that gives an immediate response. It is also appropriate if anaphylactic shock occurs to give IV fluids to maintain the circulatory volume.

1.10 D: It may have a lag period of up to 50 years between exposure and diagnosis

Mesothelioma is a malignant tumour of the pleura. It is not exclusive to those exposed to asbestos; however, the vast majority are due to this cause. Similarly, although the lion's share occur in the chest it is also is found in the peritoneum. Occupational exposure to asbestos in the UK is now heavily regulated. However, up until the late 1970s/early 1980s it was routinely used in a number of trades, including the construction and shipbuilding industries. This invariably fatal tumour demonstrates a lag period between exposure and diagnosis. The period may be up to 50 years and typically is within the 20- to 30-year range. For this reason within the UK the predicted peak of incidence of mesothelioma is 2012. The tumour is usually unilateral and frequently presents with a malignant pleural effusion. In advanced disease it may be difficult to distinguish an effusion from pleural tumour on plain CXR. The effusion will be an exudate. Diagnosis is usually by CT imaging with/without thorascopically guided biopsy. Open lung biopsy is only undertaken if other biopsy modalities are unfeasible. There is no known cure. Treatment is supportive and palliative. Five-year survival is less than 5%. The association with smoking is important. Smoking does not cause mesothelioma, however smoking and asbestos do both cause bronchial carcinoma and together they act as synergistic rather than additive risk factors for this disease.

Chest disease from asbestos exposure

Mesothelioma

Bronchial carcinoma

Asbestosis (form of lung fibrosis)

Pleural plaques

Pleural thickening

1.11 E: Give IV *N*-acetylcysteine

Paracetamol overdose can result in acute liver failure. The amount required in grams for this to occur varies between individuals but as little as 10–15 g can be sufficient. Standard paracetamol tablets are 500 mg. One has to be particularly aware of the routine combination of paracetamol in over-the-counter (OTC) medications such as Anadin-Extra®, especially in the case of a mixed tablet overdose. It is vital that if treatment is indicated it is started as early as possible based on a reliably timed plasma paracetamol level. It must be at least 4 h following ingestion. The paracetamol level may then be checked against the treatment graph (found in the 'Emergency Treatment of Poisoning' section of the *BNF*). The instigation of treatment is commenced at a lower plasma paracetamol level in the high-risk treatment group.

High-risk treatment group

Enzyme-inducing drugs (eg **carbamazepine**, phenytoin, rifampicin)

Alcoholics

Anorexic

Malnourished from other causes (eg HIV, nutritional failure)

This patient is in the high-risk treatment group due to her anti-epileptic medication. She requires treatment, although her plasma paracetamol level would not indicate treatment was necessary if she were not in this high-risk group. Activated charcoal is only useful if given within an hour of ingestion. Although both antidotes *N*-acetylcysteine and methionine are suitable it is standard procedure to use *N*-acetylcyteine as first-line treatment. These provide hepatic glutathione which is depleted in paracetamol overdose.

Treatment regime of *N*-acetylcysteine

Dosing (mg/kg)	Dilutant (IVI)	Duration	70-kg patient
150	200 ml 5% dextrose	15 min	10.5 g
50	500 ml 5% dextrose	4 h	3.5 g
100	1000 ml 5% dextrose	16 h	7 g

1.12 D: Blood film

Disseminated intravascular coagulation (DIC) = abnormal clotting and bleeding at the same time. It is a widespread disorder of clotting, caused by a variety of mechanisms, resulting in a depletion of clotting factors. A blood film will identify fragmented erythrocytes and helmet cells.

Blood Tests in DIC
- APTT ↑
- PTT ↑
- · Fibrinogen degradation products (eg, D-dimer) ↑
- Platelets ↓
- Fibrinogen ↓

Causes of DIC
- Malignancy
- Septicaemia
- Severe burns
- **Severe pre-eclampsia**
- Retained fetal products

Treatment is with replacement of blood products – packed cells, coagulation factors and platelets.

1.13 C: 3000 ml IV saline

The first action on observing an elevated calcium is to clarify whether it is a true hypercalcaemia. If the albumin value is provided and low this can be calculated simply using the equation for corrected calcium.

Corrected calcium = serum calcium + 0.02(40 – albumin)

This patient = 3.13 + 0.02(40–37) = 3.19.

The first course of action is always to ensure that the patient is adequately hydrated. A generous volume of clear intravenous fluids (3000–4000 ml of normal saline) should be administered and then the serum calcium rechecked. Although this patient is for palliative care she is symptomatic from her hypercalcaemia so simple intervention is warranted.

If her calcium remains elevated a single dose of IV bisphosphonate, such as pamidronate, may be prescribed.

1.14 A: E3V3M4

The Glasgow Coma Scale (GCS) is a routinely used and accepted method of accurately and objectively recording a patient's conscious level. It is an-easy-to use scoring system which may be recorded in a reproducible fashion by nursing or medical staff. Scored in 3 independent categories – EYE OPENING, VERBAL RESPONSE AND MOTOR RESPONSE – it is scored out of 15. Scoring should be given for the three individual categories.

Glasgow Coma Scale

Best eye response (4)	1. No eye opening
	2. Eye opening to pain
	3. Eye opening to verbal command
	4. Eyes open spontaneously
Best verbal response (5)	1. No verbal response
	2. Incomprehensible sounds
	3. Inappropriate words
	4. Confused
	5. Orientated
Best motor response (6)	1. No motor response
	2. Extension to pain
	3. Flexion to pain
	4. Withdrawal from pain
	5. Localising pain
	6. Obeys commands

It is a compulsory vital sign for head injury patients and those before and after neurosurgical intervention.

1.15 A: Fluoxetine

This man is experiencing a depressive episode of at least moderate severity. Antidepressants are indicated as part of a wider package of care. All of the above treatments are antidepressants. Fluoxetine (a selective serotonin reuptake inhibitor) is most suitable as first-line treatment because of its efficacy, patient acceptability (lower rate of side-effects) and lesser toxicity in overdose (which is particularly important in this case). Electroconvulsive therapy (ECT) is reserved for more severe depression where there is either an immediate risk to life or where other treatments have been ineffective. ECT can also be used to treat catatonia and severe and prolonged mania, although these indications are uncommon. Lithium (a salt) has anti-depressive properties, but is not a first-line treatment for unipolar depression owing to its side-effects and the necessity of blood monitoring. It is commonly used in the treatment of bipolar affective disorder.

1.16 Peptic ulceration

Answers: A B C

Duodenal ulcers do not become malignant. This is in contrast to gastric ulcers that may be malignant and must therefore be sampled by biopsy at endoscopy. Gastric ulceration is thought to be due to lowered mucosal resistance whereas duodenal ulcers are usually associated with increased acid production.

Helicobacter pylori is associated with:

- duodenal ulceration (95%)
- gastric ulceration (75%)
- chronic antral gastritis (90%).

1.17 Erythema nodosum

Answers: A B C D

Erythema nodosum is a painful rash usually occurring on the lower leg but it may also occur on the forearm. It is produced by conditions that cause a subcutaneous vasculitis. Causes include any streptococcal infection, acute sarcoidosis, tuberculosis, inflammatory bowel disease, pregnancy, leprosy, Behçet's disease and syphilis.

Drugs that may cause erythema nodosum include penicillin, oral contraceptives, codeine, salicylates and barbiturates.

1.18 Urine testing

Answers: D E

Normal urine contains <20 mg/l of albumin. A dipstick detects >150 mg/l. The level between the two is known as microalbuminuria and it is an early indicator of diabetic nephropathy.

Urine dipsticks can detect blood and the presence of white cells, but only microscopy detects casts (read the question carefully!).

Dipsticks are relatively insensitive to globulin and Bence–Jones proteins. White cells indicate inflammation/infection.

Nitrite is due to bacterial metabolism. Its absence does not exclude infection, but its presence on dipstick testing indicates infection with a specificity of 95%.

1.19 Goitre

Answers: A B C D

Pregnancy and puberty are both physiological causes of a goitre.

In Graves' disease the gland is diffusely enlarged, firm and often associated with a bruit.

Excess doses of carbimazole induce goitre.

Exogenous iodine inhibits thyroid-stimulating hormone (TSH) release and thus the stimulus for thyroid gland hypertrophy. Hence, in areas of iodine deficiency, people may develop a goitre.

Items D and E are often incorrectly answered.

1.20 Syncope   Answers: A C D E

This is a very common question and may be found in both the adult and paediatric sections. Pertussis infection causes episodes of persistent coughing and anoxia that can result in syncope.

Ménière's disease causes vertigo, tinnitus and deafness but not true syncope. Hypertrophic obstructive cardiomyopathy (HOCM) may result in such marked ventricular hypertrophy as to cause obstruction to cardiac outflow.

Always remember any arrhythmia can cause syncope.

1.21 Glycosuria   Answers: A B D E

One percent of the population has a low renal threshold for glucose. Glucocorticoids and growth hormone increase blood glucose levels and may produce hyperglycaemia. Conversely, Addison's disease may cause hypoglycaemia.

In Fanconi syndrome amino acids are also excreted in the urine due to a generalised proximal tubular defect.

Growth hormone has a diabetogenic effect.

Do not be misled by the word 'may' and mark item C as true.

1.22 Diarrhoea   Answers: A B C E

The definition of diarrhoea is the passage of loose stools in excess of 300 g in 24 h. It is useful to divide the causes into whether the stool is:

- Watery: dietary indiscretions; infections, eg cholera, rotavirus; metabolic, eg hyperthyroidism, hypocalcaemia, Addison's disease, carcinoid syndrome; diabetic autonomic neuropathy produces diarrhoea, especially nocturnal.
  Note: Addison's disease may also cause constipation, as may hypothyroidism and hypercalcaemia (hence D is false).
- Bloody: inflammatory bowel disease; bowel malignancy; infection, eg *Salmonella, Shigella, Clostridium difficile.*
- Steatorrhoea: small bowel malabsorption; pancreatic disease.

1.23 Hypercalcaemia   Answers: C E

The most common causes of hypercalcaemia are hyperparathyroidism and malignancy.

In sarcoidosis non-caseating granulomas form. These contain activated macrophages which produce a PTH-related peptide (PTH is parathyroid hormone) resulting in hypercalcaemia.

The raised calcium levels produced by sarcoidosis, multiple myeloma and vitamin D toxicity are typically steroid suppressible.

Other causes include benign familial hypercalcaemia, thyrotoxicosis, hypothyroidism in infants, phaeochromocytoma and drugs such as lithium and thiazide diuretics.

Pseudohypoparathyroidism is caused by end-organ resistance to PTH. It is associated with short stature, short metacarpals and intellectual impairment. It is called 'pseudo' because there is a biochemical picture of hypoparathyroidism with low calcium and high phosphate, although in fact the PTH is not low but is appropriately high.

Pseudopseudohypoparathyroidism is so called because it produces phenotypic features of pseudohypoparathyroidism but without calcium abnormality.

Acute pancreatitis causes hypocalcaemia because of extensive fat necrosis.

Paget's disease causes increased bone turnover. Calcium and phosphate are normal but alkaline phosphatase is elevated. However, after a period of immobilisation calcium levels may rise.

1.24 Normal chest X-ray   Answers: A B

The right hemidiaphragm is higher than the left because it is 'pushed' up by the liver.

The left hilum is higher than the right.

The right main bronchus is lower, shorter, wider and more vertical than the left and hence inhaled foreign bodies (eg peanuts) may lodge in it.

The lower end of the trachea is slightly to the right of the midline. The right lung consists of three lobes. The upper and middle lobes are anterior and are separated from each other by the horizontal fissure. The oblique fissure demarcates the lower lobe that lies posteriorly. In the left lung, only the upper (anterior) and lower (posterior) lobes are present, separated from each other by the oblique fissure.

29

Magnification of the heart occurs in an AP and a portable film. This is because the film is behind the patient's back and the X-rays shone from the front produce a wider angle to reach it.

1.25 Papilloedema   Answers: B C D E

Causes of papilloedema can be divided as follows:

- Raised intracranial pressure:
  Space-occupying lesion (tumour, cerebral abscess); benign intracranial hypertension (OCP, retinoids, tetracyclines); hypertensive encephalopathy; hypercapnia; venous sinus thrombosis
- Accelerated phase hypertension (malignant hypertension)
- Retinal vein obstruction
- Tumour; cortical venous sinus thrombosis; central retinal vein thrombosis
- Miscellaneous (rare). Metabolic: hypercapnia, vitamin A poisoning, lead poisoning. Endocrine: hypoparathyroidism, exophthalmos. Haematological: sudden/severe anaemia. Infection: subacute bacterial endocarditis.

1.26 Cystic fibrosis   Answers: C E

Cystic fibrosis is an important autosomal recessive condition which occurs in 1 in 2000 live births. The most common mutation responsible is found on the delta F508 region of chromosome 7. Screening for the carrier status is possible and prenatal diagnosis by amniocentesis is possible.

Presentation may be with bowel obstruction due to meconium ileus in babies or meconium ileus equivalent at an older age. Frequent respiratory tract infections with the development of bronchiectasis or simply a failure to thrive should lead to a suspicion of the diagnosis.

The defect is due to an abnormality of chloride ion transport and the resulting excess of sodium loss in the sweat forms the basis of the sweat test for cystic fibrosis. Many body secretions become abnormally viscous; for example, in the lung predisposing to infection, and also in the pancreas leading to malabsorption and an increased risk of diabetes mellitus. The thickened bowel secretions and steatorrhoea predispose to bowel obstruction (meconium ileus equivalent). This can be made worse by surgery and should be treated conservatively. Liver cirrhosis with portal hypertension may develop.

In the male the vas deferens is absent and so although sperm production is virtually normal its transport is not, resulting in infertility.

The mainstay of treatment is regular physiotherapy with postural drainage, early use of antibiotics during infective exacerbations, and pancreatic enzyme replacement. Nebulised DNase is of use in thinning lung secretions. Gene therapy using liposomes and viruses as vectors to carry the normal gene is at an experimental stage. Most patients survive well into adulthood.

1.27 Pulmonary embolism   Answers: A B

Other options which might occur with this question include:

- Pulsus paradoxus: true; see below
- Deep venous thrombosis: false; a DVT may cause a pulmonary embolism, but not vice versa
- Heparin treatment should only be started when a positive VQ scan result is obtained: false; see below.

Pulmonary embolism may be mild or severe, single or multiple.

Although it may be asymptomatic, it usually produces pleuritic chest pain, tachypnoea and tachycardia. The JVP may be elevated and a pulsus paradoxus may be present.

In any patient with a cough, haemoptysis or hypotension a pulmonary embolus must be considered.

Hypoxia occurs and the oxygen saturation falls. Hyperventilation produces a fall in PCO_2.

The most common ECG finding is a sinus tachycardia. Signs of right heart strain including right bundle branch block (RBBB) may also occur. The classic S1 Q3 T3 (an S wave in V1, Q wave in lead III and T wave inversion in lead III) is uncommon. The chest X-ray is often normal but a small pleural effusion may occur. Band shadows from atelectasis occur in both infection and infarction. Wedge-shaped peripheral consolidation may also occur.

If a pulmonary embolism is suspected the patient should be given heparin (providing there are no contraindications) before obtaining a ventilation/perfusion (VQ) scan. Treatment also involves giving oxygen and appropriate analgesia.

A VQ scan compares the distribution of blood flow with the parts of the lung being ventilated. When a blood clot lodges in a major blood vessel, blood is diverted from it to other vessels creating a perfusion defect. Ventilation is usually unaffected leading to a mismatched defect in ventilation and perfusion. Spiral CT with intravenous contrast using a pulmonary angiogram protocol is very sensitive in the diagnosis of a pulmonary embolus.

1.28 Dysphagia   **Answers: A B C D**

Dysphagia literally means difficulty with swallowing. It does not necessarily imply there is pain or vomiting, although these may coexist.

There may be a physical obstruction in the lumen of the oesophagus; for example, oesophageal carcinoma or a benign peptic stricture.

Disorders of the muscle wall and/or its nerve supply may also produce dysphagia, for example:

- pseudo-bulbar palsy: bilateral stroke
- bulbar palsy: motor neurone disease, Guillain–Barré syndrome, polio, myasthenia gravis
- autonomic plexus disorders: achalasia, Chagas disease, Guillain–Barré syndrome.

Anxiety may cause globus hystericus.

Pyloric stenosis produces projectile vomiting but not dysphagia.

1.29 Acromegaly   **Answers: A C D E**

Acromegaly is produced by an excess of growth hormone. Before puberty, excess growth hormone produces the syndrome of gigantism. After the epiphyses have fused an increase in height does not occur but instead there is an overgrowth of organs and soft tissue. The face is enlarged with prominent supraorbital ridges, enlarged jaw (prognathism), widely spaced teeth and poor occlusion of the teeth when the mouth closes. The tongue is large. The hands are enlarged and spade-like; they have a doughy feel to them and the skin is greasy.

The pituitary macroadenoma that is usually responsible may cause compression of the optic chiasm producing a visual field defect. This is usually a bilateral hemianopia, but an upper outer quadrantanopia may be an early sign. Optic atrophy may occur but blindness is not a common feature of acromegaly.

Other organs increase in size and hepatosplenomegaly may occur. An increase in heart size may produce a cardiomyopathy. Soft tissue overgrowth may cause compression of nerves, for example the median nerve, producing carpal tunnel syndrome. Arthropathy is also a feature. Hypertension is common and, as growth hormone causes an increase in blood glucose, diabetes mellitus may also result.

It is said that one-third of patients present because of symptoms, one-third because they notice a change in their appearance and one-third are noticed by their doctors to have a change in appearance.

Best of five and multiple choice questions – Paper 1 – Answers

The important features may be remembered as follows:

A   Arthropathy
B   Blood pressure (increase)
C   Carpal tunnel syndrome
D   Diabetes mellitus
E   Enlargement (of organs, face, hands and feet)
F   Field defect (bitemporal hemianopia).

1.30 Osteoporosis   Answers: A B C D E

Osteoporosis is a condition where a reduction in bone density occurs, predisposing to fractures. The bone constituents are normal but reduced. Serum calcium, phosphate and alkaline phosphatase are normal.

Bone formation/remodelling is dependent on normal movement, metabolic factors and hormones. Metabolic disorders, such as thyrotoxicosis, Cushing's syndrome and steroid therapy, cause this reduction in bone mass.

Oestrogen promotes bone growth, and deficiency states, such as the menopause, are important risk factors. Hormone replacement therapy (HRT) not only prevents further bone loss but can promote bone regeneration. However due to concerns regarding an increased risk of breast cancer, HRT is not recommended as first-line treatment for osteoporosis in postmenopausal women. In prolonged immobilisation the local stress/strain on bone is absent; remodelling does not occur, increasing the risk of osteoporosis. A low body weight, for example in athletes and those with anorexia nervosa, also predisposes to it and genetic and racial factors are important. (Asians and Orientals have a higher incidence.) The incidence also rises with age and is more common in women; by the age of 70 a woman will have lost 50% of her bone mass and one in two women will have sustained an osteoporotic fracture.

1.31 Ocular complications of diabetes mellitus   Answers: C D E

The most common form of diabetic eye disease is diabetic retinopathy which is classified as follows:

- Background retinopathy
  (1) Dot haemorrhages which are actually capillary microaneurysms
  (2) Blot haemorrhages which are caused by leakage of blood into the deeper layers of the retina
  (3) Hard exudates which are bright yellow/white clearly defined lesions caused by exudates of lipid and protein. These changes take at least 10 years to develop.

33

- Maculopathy
- More commonly seen in non-insulin-dependent diabetes mellitus (NIDDM). Hard exudates appear in a circular pattern around the macula; a serious complication, as visual acuity may decline rapidly.
- Pre-proliferative retinopathy
  The following are classified as pre-proliferative changes as they are thought to induce proliferative changes:
  (1) Cotton wool spots (soft exudates) which are patches of retinal oedema caused by ischaemia
  (2) Venous beading/looping
  (3) More than three blot haemorrhages
- Proliferative retinopathy
  Hypoxia is thought to be the signal for new vessel formation. These new vessels are fragile and haemorrhage easily. This encourages fibrous proliferation producing traction bands and eventually retinal detachment. Fifty per cent of these patients will be blind in 5 years.
- Cataracts
  More common with advancing age; juvenile/snowflake cataracts are diffuse, rapidly progressive cataracts associated with poorly controlled diabetes mellitus
- Glaucoma
  Diabetics have an increased risk of acute glaucoma due to rubeosis iridis (new vessel formation at the iris blocks fluid drainage at the canal of Schlemm leading to a sudden increase in intraocular pressure). There is also an increased incidence of chronic glaucoma
- Cranial nerve palsy – especially III.

1.32 Primary hyperaldosteronism　　　　　　　　　**Answers: A B**

This question requires a knowledge of the biochemistry of primary hyperaldosteronism:

BP
Na renin (kidneys)
Angiotensinogen (liver)

Angiotensin I (lungs)

Angiotensin II
Vasoconstriction
Aldosterone (adrenal glands)

Acts on distal renal tubule

Na retention hypertension
Decreased K^+
Decreased H^+

Aldosterone increases sodium reabsorption in exchange for potassium and hydrogen in the distal renal tubule, resulting in a hypernatraemic hypokalaemic metabolic alkalosis.

Renin levels are low because of negative feedback by increased aldosterone.

Salt and water retention produce hypertension.

1.33 Insulin-dependent diabetes mellitus   Answer: C

Diabetic nephropathy affects 25–30% of diabetic patients. Patients with diabetic renal disease will almost certainly also have some degree of retinopathy, but the converse is not true. Diabetic retinopathy is much more common than nephropathy.

Maculopathy is more common in type II diabetes mellitus.

Pre-proliferative and proliferative retinopathy is most commonly found in type I diabetes mellitus.

The aetiology of diabetes mellitus is complex. An increased susceptibility may be inherited, with the greatest risk if the father is diabetic.

Ninety-five per cent of insulin-dependent diabetes mellitus (IDDM) patients carry HLA DR3, HLA DR4 or both.
Interestingly, people with HLA DR2 have a reduced risk.
Viruses – *Coxsackie type B4*.

The main problem in type I diabetes is a lack of insulin, whereas in type II insulin is present but there is a peripheral resistance to it. During illness the stress hormones (eg cortisol) increase, causing hyperglycaemia and increasing insulin requirements.

1.34 Nephrotic syndrome   Answers: A B E

The definition of nephrotic syndrome comprises:

● proteinuria of 3–5 g over 24 h
● hypoalbuminuria
● peripheral oedema.

It is also associated with a hypercoagulable state and hypercholesterolaemia but this is not strictly in the formal definition. There are many causes:

- Congenital
- Acquired:
  Glomerulonephritis (most commonly minimal change, focal sclerosing, membranous)
  Diabetes
  Systemic vasculitis, especially SLE drugs (eg gold, penicillamine)
  Infection (eg malaria)
  Myeloma
  Allergies.

Interstitial nephritis, as the name implies, causes a nephritis rather than a nephrotic syndrome. Nephritis produces much less proteinuria and causes haematuria that is usually microscopic.

This question appears frequently. Other options to bear in mind are renal papillary necrosis, chronic tubulointerstitial nephritis, renal TB and polycystic renal disease. All may cause proteinuria but not enough to cause the syndrome that – remember – has a strict definition.

1.35 Paget's disease   Answer: D

In Paget's disease there is increased resorption of bone due to increased osteoclastic activity and secondary abnormal bone formation. Patients may be remarkably asymptomatic despite extensive skeletal involvement. Clinical features include bone pain and local tenderness, bone deformity and fractures. The skull is enlarged and the bony overgrowth may produce cranial nerve damage; for example, optic atrophy and deafness. The latter may also be caused by overgrowth of the ossicles. High output cardiac failure may occur and although everyone remembers the complication of osteosarcoma, note that it only occurs in 1–2% of patients. Remember the mnemonic **PANICS:**

Pain
Arthritis
Nerve compression
Increased bone size
Cardiac failure
Sarcoma

Diagnosis is made by history, examination and investigations.

Bone turnover is increased resulting in a raised alkaline phosphatase. Although bone is resorbed it is also re-formed and so serum calcium and phosphate are normal (recent immobilisation may cause hypercalcaemia).

Radiography show disorganised bone, with bony expansion and a coarsened trabecular pattern. Treatment includes pain relief, calcitonin, sodium etidronate and treatment of complications.

1.36 Diabetes mellitus   Answer: A

This is a very difficult question. Remember the WHO criteria for the diagnosis of diabetes mellitus:

	Fasting glucose (mmol/l)	Random glucose (mmol/l)
Plasma	>7.8	>11.1
Whole blood	>6.7	>10.0

Whole blood values are 1.1 mmol/l less than plasma because the red blood cells use up glucose. Ideally, two abnormal values should be obtained. When a value between 7.8 and 11.1 mmol/l or between 6.7 and 10 mmol/l occurs then a 75-g glucose tolerance test should be performed. A fasting plasma glucose ≥7.8 mmol/l or a 2-h value ≥1.1 mmol/l is diagnostic. Values in between imply impaired glucose tolerance, and a proportion of these people will go on to develop diabetes mellitus.

Islet cell antibodies are of interest because they provide evidence for an autoimmune aetiology, but they are not currently used in routine diagnosis.

Glycosuria reflects the degree of diabetic control, but 1% of the population and pregnant women have a low renal threshold for glucose reabsorption and so glycosuria is suggestive of diabetes mellitus but is not diagnostic. Retinal new vessel formation occurs in response to hypoxia of any aetiology, for example sickle cell disease.

1.37 Ptosis   Answers: A B E

A ptosis is a drooping eyelid and may be complete (the eye is closed) or partial. It may be unilateral or bilateral.

Damage at any of the following sites will result in a ptosis:

- III nerve damage: posterior communicating artery aneurysm, midbrain lesion.
- Sympathetic nerve damage: Horner's syndrome.
- Muscle/neuromuscular nerve junction: dystrophia myotonica (usually bilateral), myasthenia gravis (ptosis is fatigable and often bilateral).

Parasympathetic damage itself does not cause a ptosis. See Paper 1, Question 1.47 on pupil dilation for details.

Note that a VII nerve palsy results in an inability to close the eye. *It never causes a ptosis.*

1.38 Bell's palsy   Answers: A B C

A Bell's palsy is a common, acute, isolated facial nerve palsy. Damage to the nerve occurs in the petrous part of the temporal bone, ie before the branch to the stapedius muscle is given off. Stapedius is protective against noise and so temporary damage to its nerve supply results in hyperacusis. Deafness is not a feature.

The patient often complains of pain behind the ear at the onset, marked unilateral facial weakness and sometimes loss of taste.

Ptosis does not occur. In fact, the opposite occurs; the eye may not close, leading to chemosis and ulceration.

1.39 Acute myocardial infarction   Answers: A B C D E

Myocardial infarction may present with the characteristic features of severe crushing central chest pain, palpitations and nausea; but often, particularly in elderly people, symptoms are less specific or even absent. Patients presenting with injury from a fall must have the cause of the fall looked at; it may be due to an arrhythmia caused by myocardial infarction. Myocardial infarction may precipitate an acute confusional state, particularly in elderly people. In diabetic patients, a myocardial infarction may precipitate hyperglycaemia or even be silent.

Peri- or post-operative infarction may pass unnoticed until oliguria is detected. Although post-operative oliguria has many causes, for example blood loss or dehydration, it is worth remembering that a myocardial infarction may produce a fall in cardiac output and hence oliguria.

1.40 Finger clubbing   Answers: A E

All cyanotic congenital heart disease can cause finger clubbing; for example, transposition of the great vessels and Fallot's tetralogy. The important point is that there must be a right to left shunt. An atrial septal defect (ASD) and small ventricular septal defect (VSD; for example, maladie de Roger) do not produce cyanosis unless complicated by Eisenmenger's syndrome, which is not mentioned in the question. Rheumatic fever does not cause clubbing but remember that subacute bacterial endocarditis can.

1.41 Cardiac arrest   Answers: B C

Many surveys of cardiopulmonary resuscitation have shown that most junior doctors are unsafe! Recently medical schools and hospitals have improved their requirements for cardiopulmonary resuscitation (CPR) training. Numerous questions have been set for the MRCP and OSCE examinations.

The most common cause of a cardiac arrest is ventricular fibrillation. The single lifesaving treatment is DC cardioversion and the earlier this is given the better the chance of survival. If a delay is likely, airway management and cardiac massage must be started until defibrillation is possible. Cardiac massage involves sternal compression to 4–5 cm (1.5–2 in) at a rate of 30 compressions to 2 rescue breaths whether one or two people are present. Note that this is a change from the previous guidelines of 15 compressions to 2 breaths. (Note: the guidelines change frequently!)

The other types of cardiac arrest are asystole where QRS complexes are absent and electromechanical dissociation (EMD), ie the electrical activity of the heart is no longer accompanied by mechanical activity and as a result there is no cardiac output. The important causes of EMD are:

- The four H's: hypovolaemia, hypothermia, hypocalcaemia and hypoxia
- The four T's: cardiac tamponade, pulmonary thromboembolism, tension pneumothorax and toxic/therapeutic disturbances.

Calcium chloride, therefore, is recommended in the management of EMD but not asystole. Asystole is difficult to treat. In the European protocol DC cardioversion is recommended in cases where ventricular fibrillation cannot be excluded; atropine is given, which blocks the inhibitory effect of the vagus nerve. If QRS complexes then appear, pacing is necessary. The prognosis is poor.

1.42 Autoantibodies   Answers: B C D

- Liver disease: primary biliary cirrhosis – antimitochondrial antibody and antinuclear factor (also raised IgM); chronic active hepatitis – anti-smooth muscle antibody (also raised IgG); alcoholic liver disease – no specific antibodies but raised IgA.
- Connective tissue disease: SLE – anti-dsDNA (anti-double-stranded DNA is highly specific for SLE); anti-Sm (note this is not the same as anti-smooth muscle antibody – Sm refers to Smith, the person who discovered the antibody); anti-Ro – associated with heart block in neonates whose mothers have this antibody); anti-La.
- Systemic sclerosis: anti-Scl 70 anti-centromere in the CREST variant.

- Polymyositis: anti-Jo.
- Sjögren's: rheumatoid factor, anti-Ro, anti-La.
- Rheumatoid arthritis: rheumatoid factor [this is IgM antibody against the Fc portion of IgG. It is not specific for rheumatoid (Rh) arthritis; 30% of patients with SLE and 90% of patients with Sjögren's have Rh factor. It also occurs in sarcoid and any condition that stimulates IgG production. Although the Rh factor titre correlates with disease activity, some patients with Rh arthritis never develop the antibody].

1.43 Chronic obstructive pulmonary disease   **Answers: A B**

- Chronic obstructive pulmonary disease (COPD). This term is used to describe chronic bronchitis, emphysema and the spectrum that exists between them. Most people with COPD have a mixture of the two conditions.
- Chronic bronchitis. The definition is clinical. The essential feature is a cough productive of sputum for 3 months of the year, for 2 or more consecutive years.

Pathology – there is mucus gland hypertrophy and the bronchial walls become inflamed; they undergo squamous metaplasia and fibrous changes.

Clinical features include dyspnoea and a productive cough. On examination the patient breathes with pursed lips, the chest is hyper-inflated, the crico-sternal distance is reduced and accessory muscles of respiration may be in use. The term **blue bloater** describes a patient who hypoventilates and retains carbon dioxide. Stimulation of ventilation depends on the hypoxic drive and so oxygen must be used with care. Consequences of hypoxia include:

- cyanosis (hence the term blue)
- polycythaemia because of hypoxic stimulation of erythropoietin production by the kidney (in fact, venesection may be of benefit)
- changes to pulmonary blood vessels resulting in pulmonary hypertension and cor pulmonale.

The **pink puffer** patient is less hypoxic and the patient hyperventilates in an attempt to correct poor gaseous exchange. Such patients often tolerate >24% oxygen. It used to be thought that a blue bloater had chronic bronchitis and the pink puffer had emphysema, but post-mortem studies have not supported this. Obese patients with COPD are more likely to develop the blue-bloater-type of picture as obesity increases the risk of hypoventilation. Use the terms with care – some examiners like using them, but others dislike it.

Management of acute attack:

- ABC – management of the airway, breathing and circulation
- IV access and send blood for full blood count (FBC), urea and electrolytes (U&Es), blood cultures
- Arterial blood gases
- Controlled oxygen, ie 24% oxygen increased if PCO_2 allows
- Steroids – IV hydrocortisone or oral prednisolone
- Antibiotics – infected exacerbations are most likely to be due to *Haemophilus influenzae* and are treated with amoxicillin or trimethoprim or IV antibiotics if indicated
- Beta-2 agonists (eg salbutamol) given as nebuliser. Anticholinergics (eg ipratropium bromide) can also be given
- Physiotherapy to expel secretions
- Consider respiratory stimulants, such as doxapram
- Nasal ventilation or intubation and ventilation if clinically indicated.

Long-term management:

- Stop smoking
- Drugs, for example inhaled beta-2 stimulants, anticholinergics, steroids
- Home oxygen – this should be considered for patients with severe symptoms. There have been two major trials which show that 2 l/min of oxygen to maintain an oxygen saturation of >90% for 15 h per day improves the symptoms. An increase to 19 h maximum per day actually decreases mortality. Patients must have stopped smoking
- Yearly flu vaccine (provided there are no contraindications).

1.44 Rib fracture   Answers: A B C E

Spontaneous rib fractures may occur in the absence of trauma when there is an abnormality of the rib. This may be due to osteoporosis, primary lung tumour or metastatic disease. Tumours that spread to bone include breast, lung, thyroid, kidney and prostate. Trauma may obviously cause a rib fracture but coughing, especially in elderly people, may be sufficient to cause several fractures. A rib fracture may cause a pneumothorax but not vice versa.

1.45 Rapid respiration   Answers: A B D E

The cerebral cortex influences the respiratory rate; for example, anxiety increases the respiratory rate via increased sympathetic nervous activity. The respiratory centre in the pons responds to decreases in pH, increased H^+, increased PCO_2 and decreased PO_2 by increasing the respiratory rate. Drugs such as doxapram and aspirin in overdose can also stimulate the respiratory centre, whereas drugs such as opiates and sedatives cause hypoventilation. The pons is also influenced by peripheral chemoreceptors.

In diabetic ketoacidosis it is not the glucose level itself but the fall in pH that stimulates respiration. In uncomplicated hypoglycaemia there is no change in pH.

1.46 Pleural effusion   Answers: A B D E

Causes of a pleural effusion can be classified according to the size of the effusion or the protein content, for example:

Size:

- Large: neoplastic especially lung, breast, mesothelioma, infection (eg TB), trauma
- Moderate: pneumonia, heart failure
- Small: pulmonary embolism, pneumonia, heart failure, pancreatitis, subphrenic abscess, connective tissue disease

Protein content:

- Transudate (protein <30 g/l): heart failure, liver cirrhosis, nephrotic syndrome, Meigs' syndrome
- Exudate (protein >30 g/l): malignancy (may be blood-stained), infection, pulmonary embolism, trauma, rheumatoid arthritis (glucose content very low, rheumatoid factor high), C3, C4 (complement components) present, subphrenic abscess (this is most common on the left side), pancreatitis (high amylase levels in the effusion).

Retroperitoneal fibrosis does not cause a pleural effusion.

1.47 Pupil dilatation   Answer: A

Parasympathetic nerve fibres and fibres from the convergence centre pass via the third nerve to the pupil, resulting in pupil constriction. Sympathetic nerve stimulation causes pupil dilation. The pupil becomes smaller with age. Item C really did feature in a previous paper.

1.48 Spontaneous pneumothorax   Answers: A C

Spontaneous pneumothorax is the sudden entry of air into a pleural space (ie the space between the visceral and the parietal pleura) and the subsequent collapse of the underlying lung. It occurs six times more commonly in men than in women. Symptoms range from mild pleuritic chest pain to respiratory compromise.

Investigations include a chest X-ray (NB if a tension pneumothorax is suspected this should be treated immediately even before a chest X-ray is requested). The chest X-ray confirms the diagnosis, demonstrates the presence of significant fluid levels and is used to assess the degree of collapse.

- Small pneumothorax: a rim of air is present around the lung
- Moderate-sized pneumothorax: collapse halfway to the heart border
- Complete pneumothorax: airless lung separated from the diaphragm.

Treatment depends on the individual patient and varies according to symptoms, the degree of collapse and whether there is underlying lung disease or bleeding. Patients should be admitted if the pneumothorax is the result of trauma or if there is underlying lung disease. Patients should also be admitted if they are symptomatic, ie pain is persisting or increasing or there is shortness of breath on slow walking. Patients should also be admitted if the X-ray shows a complete collapse or a fluid level is present in the costophrenic angle.

Aspiration is easy to perform. It causes minimal discomfort to the patient. Consequently, it has become a more popular treatment than intercostal tube insertion in recent years. In fact, the British Thoracic Society now recommends aspiration as the treatment of choice even in a 100% pneumothorax, ie complete collapse of the lung. If aspiration is not successful then intercostal drainage tube insertion is required. For guidance of chest drain insertion see question 4.42, Paper 4. The reabsorption rate after a pneumothorax that is not treated is 1.25%/day – so a total pneumothorax would take 80 days!

1.49 Sarcoidosis   **Answers: A B C D E**

Sarcoidosis is a multisystem disorder. Abnormal blood investigations include a cytopenia, occasionally eosinophilia, raised ACE, raised erythrocyte sedimentation rate (ESR) and hypercalcaemia.

Respiratory system abnormalities are manifested by:

- chest X-ray changes, eg upper/mid zone fibrosis; bilateral hilar lymphadenopathy
- decreased lung volumes
- reduced diffusing capacity (KCO); normal FEV_1/FVC ratio
- blood gases may show mild hypoxia
- ^{67}gallium lung scan shows increased uptake
- bronchoscopy and transbronchial biopsies or lymph node biopsies show non-caseating granulomas.

1.50 Urinary tract infection Answers: A B C

This is a very common question. It is designed to illustrate the non-specific, often vague symptoms that an infection may produce in elderly people, but also to warn that some symptoms are more sinister and need to be investigated thoroughly.

Any infection can produce an acute confusional state, especially in elderly people. Urinary frequency, urgency and incontinence are common symptoms, as is haematuria, but not enough to cause anaemia that should be investigated. Wandering at night is a feature of dementia.

1.51 Portosystemic encephalography Answers: A C D E

Liver cirrhosis causes portal hypertension and this high pressure in the portal system opens up anastomoses with the systemic circulation. Normally toxic substances absorbed from the gut are carried in the portal circulation and broken down by the liver but now these reach the systemic circulation via the anastomoses and hence act on the brain to cause encephalopathy.

Electrolyte abnormalities and drugs that provoke them, for example diuretics, worsen encephalopathy. The brain is also exquisitely sensitive to the effects of drugs acting on the CNS, for example opiates and benzodiazepines, which are normally metabolised by the liver.

Patients are at risk of developing oesophageal varices and consequently GI bleed. The proteins from the blood are not broken down by the liver in the normal way and these nitrogenous products are also toxic to the brain.

Bacteria in the bowel also produce nitrogenous products and if these are allowed to accumulate, for example due to constipation, encephalopathy may be precipitated. Treatment involves correcting the underlying cause, ie stopping offending drugs, correcting electrolyte disturbances, and lactulose and enemas to clear the bowel. Oral neomycin used to be used to sterilise the gut, but it was found that it encouraged the growth of harmful nitrogen-metabolising bacteria at the expense of useful sugar-fermenting bacteria.

General supportive care is the mainstay of management – prevention of GI bleed with attention to position to prevent aspiration, pressure sores, state of hydration, etc.

1.52 Arterial blood pressure Answers: B C D E

This is a difficult but important question. Normally the systolic BP falls slightly on standing (<20 mmHg) and the diastolic rises slightly (>10 mmHg).

A fall in systolic BP >20 mmHg or a diastolic fall ≥10 mmHg (remember the diastolic normally rises) is, by definition, postural hypotension and occurs with hypovolaemia and conditions producing autonomic dysfunction, such as diabetes mellitus, Guillain-Barré, and Shy-Drager syndromes.

The heart rate rises on standing and on exercise and these are also useful tests of autonomic function. Exercise also increases the arterial blood pressure but in the long term regular exercise lowers the blood pressure and pulse rate. There is a diurnal variation in the blood pressure – it is higher during the day.

Up to 10 mmHg difference between the right and left brachial pressures is normal. Any more than this is suggestive of aortic dissection, or if the blood pressure is elevated, coarctation of the aorta, with a stenosis proximal to the origin of the left subclavian artery.

When a small cuff is used a higher pressure is required to occlude the artery and hence the BP reading is falsely high.

1.53 Collapsing pulse   Answers: A B E

A large volume pulse with a brisk rise and fall is known as a collapsing pulse. It is found in high cardiac output states, for example anaemia, thyrotoxicosis, fever, aortic regurgitation and patent ductus arteriosus.

Cardiac output = stroke volume × heart rate, so if the heart rate falls the stroke volume increases to maintain the cardiac output. Bradycardia therefore causes a large volume pulse but it is not collapsing in nature. Mitral stenosis causes a reduction in cardiac output and is associated with a low volume pulse.

1.54 Mortality rates   Answers: A E

- The **maternal mortality rate** is the number of deaths of mothers attributable to pregnancy or delivery divided by the number of births.
- The **infant mortality rate** is the number of deaths in the first year of life divided by the number of live births. It is expressed per thousand live births.
- The **neonatal mortality rate** is the number of deaths in the first four weeks of life divided by the number of live births. It is also expressed per thousand live births.
- The **perinatal mortality rate** is the number of stillbirths and deaths in the first week of life, divided by the total number of births (ie live and dead). It is quoted per thousand births.

- The **stillbirth rate** is the number of stillbirths divided by the total number of births (both live and stillbirth). A stillbirth is a baby born dead after 28 weeks' gestation.

1.55 Infectious diseases   Answers: A B E

In 1992 the *Haemophilus influenzae B* vaccine (Hib) was introduced. Since then *Haemophilus influenzae* meningitis, epiglottitis and other serious infections with this organism have virtually disappeared from paediatric wards.

In 1994, measles, mumps and rubella (MMR) vaccination was administered to prevent the predicted epidemic of measles in schoolchildren. The immunisation covered over 8 million children and a reduction in the number of cases of measles occurred. However, in the late 1990s a link between MMR and autism was suggested. This link has never been proven and many studies have been performed which do not confirm the link. However, parents have become so concerned that many have chosen not to have their children vaccinated and in 2001 several cases of measles in school children were confirmed.

Smallpox was declared to have been eradicated from the world in 1980 by the World Health Organisation. The last naturally occurring case of smallpox was in Somalia in 1977. The last epidemic of smallpox in London was at the end of the nineteenth century.

Influenza A viruses are antigenically labile due to changes in the surface antigen haemagglutinin (H) and neuraminidase (N). Minor changes (so-called antigenic drift) occur from season to season. Major changes (ie antigenic shift) occur due to acquisition of a new haemagglutinin.

Influenza B may undergo minor changes (less frequently than influenza A) and does not undergo major changes.

1.56 Immunisation   Answers: B C E

The spread of infectious disease may be reduced by social factors; for example, improvement in living conditions, better sanitation, hygiene, knowledge of spread of infections, laws governing food preparation and storage. These have had a major impact on reducing the incidence of TB, typhoid and cholera. TB spreads more rapidly where there is overcrowding, poor nutrition and poverty. Cholera is spread by water contamination and typhoid is spread by food contamination.

Vaccination is largely responsible for the decline in mortality from measles, whooping cough and diphtheria.

1.57 Inhaled steroids   Answers: B C E

This is a difficult question and is more likely to come up as a single item rather than as a whole question.

Inhaled steroids may be low dose or high dose. There is concern regarding the safety of the latter. High-dose inhaled steroids can cause adrenal suppression but this is minimal. Cushing's syndrome and cataracts are not caused by inhaled steroids even at the highest doses.

Oral candidiasis and possible laryngeal myopathy are caused by low-dose inhaled steroids and are responsible for the hoarse voice often experienced by patients.

Dysphagia caused by oesophageal candidiasis can occur with the higher dose of inhaled steroids.

1.58 Polyuria   Answers: A B D

This is a very common question. It refers to an increase in the amount of urine produced, irrespective of frequency of micturition.

Antidiuretic hormone (ADH) regulates the amount of water excretion depending on plasma osmolarity. ADH acts on the distal convoluted tubule making it permeable to water and hence promoting water reabsorption. ADH deficiency or end-organ resistance to its effects will produce polyuria, for example diabetes insipidus (cranial and nephrogenic).

The solute load through the renal tubules also determines water excretion. In diabetes mellitus there is an increased glucose load. The excess glucose inside the tubules cannot be reabsorbed (the tubular maximum for absorption has been exceeded) and the glucose is excreted in the urine. Water is retained with the glucose inside the tubules to maintain iso-osmolarity and so excess water is excreted as well as glucose. This results in polyuria and polydipsia, typical symptoms of diabetes mellitus.

Chronic hypokalaemia and hypercalcaemia damage the renal tubules producing resistance to ADH and hence polyuria.

In chronic renal failure, tubular dysfunction may result in polyuria.

An epileptic fit may cause urinary incontinence, but not polyuria.

Psychogenic causes should also be remembered, for example compulsive water drinking, which is more common in schizophrenics.

You may be asked about supraventricular tachycardia (SVT) – the answer to this is true because atrial arrhythmias stimulate atrial natriuretic peptide, which causes a diuresis.

1.59 Systolic murmurs   Answers: B C D

In general, systolic murmurs are mid- or late systolic, whereas diastolic murmurs are early or mid-diastolic. Aortic stenosis and pulmonary stenosis produce ejection mid-systolic murmurs. Mitral valve prolapse usually produces a late systolic murmur best heard at the apex. Other causes of a late systolic murmur include coarctation of the aorta and hypertrophic obstructive cardiomyopathy (HOCM). The murmur of HOCM is louder on squatting and standing.

The murmur of a VSD is best heard at the left sternal edge. Note that a very small VSD may produce a short murmur because contraction of the ventricle closes the defect early in systole.

The ejection systolic murmur heard with an ASD is actually due to a pulmonary murmur rather than the ASD itself.

1.60 Leucocytes in urine   Answers: A B C

Leucocytes in the urine occur with:

- a bacterial or chemical cystitis
- urethritis
- prostatitis
- pyelitis
- TB infection of the renal tract
- analgesic nephropathy
- renal stones.

BEST OF FIVE AND MULTIPLE CHOICE QUESTIONS PAPER 2

60 questions: time allowed 2½ hours

Best of Five Questions
Mark your answers with a tick (True) in the box provided.

2.1   A 72-year-old lady is admitted with UTI and treated with a
       cephalosporin antibiotic following microbiological advice. Two
       days later she develops green, foul-smelling diarrhoea. On
       examination her abdomen is mildly distended. Stool serology is
       positive for *Clostridium difficile*. What is the most appropriate
       treatment in the first instance?

❏   A   Observation and rehydration
❏   B   Commence oral vancomycin
❏   C   Commence oral metronidazole
❏   D   Stop cephalosporin and commence loperamide
❏   E   Commence ciprofloxacin

2.2   A 54-year-old diabetic lady is admitted with malaise by her GP.
       Liver function tests (LFTs) were taken by her GP: bilirubin
       41 μmol/l, AST 46 iu/l, ALT 56 iu/l, GGT 241 iu/l, ALP 198 iu/l.
       On examination: abdomen soft, non-tender. No palpable masses
       or organomegaly. Which one of the following is the next best
       investigation?

❏   A   CT scan abdomen
❏   B   ERCP (endoscopic retrograde cholangiopancreatography)
❏   C   Autoantibody screen
❏   D   Ultrasound scan of the abdomen
❏   E   PABA test

2.3 A 21-year-old semi-professional rugby player is admitted with a red, hot swollen left knee. No trauma has occurred. On examination: temperature 38.1°C, large left knee effusion, unable to fully extend left knee. The clinical suspicion is of a septic arthritis. What is the most likely causative organism?

❏ A *Mycobacterium tuberculosis*
❏ B *Staphylococcus aureus*
❏ C *Neisseria gonorrhoeae*
❏ D *Streptococcus viridans*
❏ E *Salmonella typhi*

2.4 A 63-year-old woman is diagnosed at bronchoscopy with a non-small-cell bronchial carcinoma. She is otherwise in good health. Staging CT imaging did not reveal any evidence of metastatic disease. Her surgeon has offered a pneumonectomy but wishes for positron emission tomography (PET) to be undertaken. How does this best further assist in patient management?

❏ A Identifies blood supply to the tumour
❏ B Locates more accurately the primary tumour mass
❏ C Labels the tumour for easier identification at surgery
❏ D Demonstrates any metastatic disease not found at CT
❏ E Shrinks the tumour mass prior to surgery

2.5 A 35-year-old man who lives in a local hostel for the homeless is added onto the medical take following a seizure. He last consumed alcohol 32 h previously and when assessed he is tremulous and anxious, wishing to self-discharge. His nutritional status and personal hygiene is poor. Which one of the following is the most essential to be carefully monitored whilst an inpatient?

❏ A GGT
❏ B Serum alcohol level
❏ C Sodium
❏ D Phosphate
❏ E Haemoglobin

2.6 A 55-year-old gentleman attends cardiology outpatients having been lost to follow-up for 2 years. He has an extensive cardiac history with two previous myocardial infarcts (MIs), peripheral vascular disease and three transient ischaemic attacks (TIAs). He is a non-insulin-dependent diabetic. Examination findings demonstrate a jugular venous pressure (JVP) raised by 2 cm, peripheral pitting oedema to the mid calf bilaterally and bilateral basal fine inspiratory crepitations. His last echocardiogram (ECHO) 3 years ago demonstrated moderately impaired left ventricular (LV) function, and mitral regurgitation. His current medications include: bisoprolol, aspirin, simvastatin, frusemide, ramipril and glicazide. Which one of the following medications if added would be of prognostic benefit?

- ❑ A Nifedipine
- ❑ B Sotalol
- ❑ C Digoxin
- ❑ D Naftidrofuryl
- ❑ E Spironolactone

2.7 A 67-year-old retired caretaker with a well documented history of COPD is admitted for his 4th time this year with shortness of breath and cough productive of green sputum. Examination findings are: respiratory rate (RR) 32 bpm, temp 37.4°C, SpO_2 86%, respiratory flap and coarse crepitations at the left base. CXR confirms left basal consolidation. Which arterial blood gas (ABG) picture is likely to belong to the above patient?

- ❑ A pH: 7.27, PaO_2: 7.1, PCO_2: 8.9, HCO_3^-: 33.20, BE –4.9 mmol
- ❑ B pH: 7.28, PaO_2: 10.4, PCO_2: 6.4, HCO_3^-: 17.95, BE –5.8 mmol
- ❑ C pH: 7.35, PaO_2: 9.0, PCO_2: 3.8, HCO_3^-: 21.90, BE +1.4 mmol
- ❑ D pH: 7.47, PaO_2: 9.6, PCO_2: 3.5, HCO_3^-: 27.40, BE +3.0 mmol
- ❑ E pH: 7.33, PaO_2: 12.8, PCO_2: 5.4, HCO_3^-: 21.80, BE –4.0 mmol

2.8 A 21-year-old sportsman attends Casualty acutely short of breath accompanied by right-sided pleuritic chest discomfort. His only past medical history is of childhood asthma and a collapsed lung aged 17 years of age. On examination – RR 16 bpm, SpO_2 95%. CXR: right-sided pneumothorax – 30% loss of lung volume. What is the most suitable course of action?

❑ A   Needle aspiration
❑ B   Chest drain placement
❑ C   Needle aspiration followed by chest drain insertion
❑ D   Observation and daily CXR
❑ E   Refer to thoracic surgeons for pleurodesis

2.9 **A 36-year-old spinster with a 10-year history of rheumatoid disease is admitted with a 'flare'. She is well known to the ward and has previously taken methotrexate, gold and sulphasalazine. The last two medications were beneficial for the first 2 years but then became less helpful even at higher doses. She is currently on oral steroids. On examination: active synovitis in eight small joints of the hands and the left wrist. Which is the next best treatment for this patient?**

❑ A   Maintain on steroids and add a bisphosphonate
❑ B   Commence leflunomide
❑ C   Use methotrexate/leflunomide combination
❑ D   Commence penicillamine
❑ E   Enrol in biological therapy programme

2.10 **A 49-year-old man is admitted with an ischaemic left leg which is unviable and requires amputation. He becomes increasing unwell whilst awaiting surgery, including experiencing breathing difficulties. An ABG was taken. pH 7.23, PO_2 12.4, PCO_2 x, HCO_3^- x. Lactate 10.3 mmol/l. What are the most likely PCO_2 and HCO_3^-?**

❑ A PCO_2 5.4 + HCO_3^- 17.4
❑ B PCO_2 4.1 + HCO_3^- 34.4
❑ C PCO_2 2.5 + HCO_3^- 34.5
❑ D PCO_2 3.8 + HCO_3^- 22.3
❑ E PCO_2 2.5 + HCO_3^- 17.5

2.11   A 72-year-old former miner is referred to the psycho-geriatrician by his GP. His daughter is concerned over his increasingly poor memory and difficulty looking after himself in the last month. Two years previously he was well and an active member of the local Rotary club. His past medical history includes an MI aged 68 years, osteoarthritis of the knees and peripheral vascular disease. On examination: bi-basal fine inspiratory crepitations. Right inguinal hernia. Left renal bruit. What is the most likely cause of this patient's symptoms?

- ❏ A   Pick's disease
- ❏ B   Alzheimer's disease
- ❏ C   Normal pressure hydrocephalus
- ❏ D   Sporadic Creutzfeldt–Jakob disease
- ❏ E   Multi-infarct dementia

2.12   A 71-year-old retired plumber is admitted with progressive shortness of breath, haemoptysis and weight loss. He is a smoker of 25 pack years. On CXR a focal mass is seen peripherally in the left lower lobe. His serum biochemistry is shown. Na^+ 136 mmol/l, K^+ 3.8 mmol/l, calcium 3.32 mmol/l, Ur 6.8 mmol/l, Cr 76 µmol/l, Alb 38 g/l. What is the most likely diagnosis?

- ❏ A   Alveolar cell bronchial carcinoma
- ❏ B   Mesothelioma
- ❏ C   Tuberculosis
- ❏ D   Squamous cell bronchial carcinoma
- ❏ E   Small (oat) cell bronchial carcinoma

2.13   A 41-year-old housewife attends neurology outpatients with a complaint of altered vision. Fundoscopy is performed and is normal. There is a full range of eye movement on examination. Visual field testing by confrontation suggests a left-sided homonymous hemianopia which is confirmed on formal perimetry tests. Where in the visual pathway is the lesion causing this field defect?

- ❏ A   Left optic tract
- ❏ B   Right optic tract
- ❏ C   Optic chiasm
- ❏ D   Left occipital lobe
- ❏ E   Right occipital lobe

2.14 A 33-year-old AIDS sufferer is admitted unwell, pyrexic and short of breath. Your senior colleague is concerned this patient has *Pneumocystis carinii* pneumonia (PCP). Which one of the following clinical findings is typical of this condition?

- ❏ A Cavitating lesions on CXR
- ❏ B Exercise desaturation
- ❏ C Presence of cervical lymphadenopathy
- ❏ D Accompanying colourless frothy sputum
- ❏ E An obstructive pattern of pulmonary function tests (PFTs)

2.15 A 24-year old man is admitted to your psychiatric ward in a state of distress saying that he knows for certain that his colleagues are plotting to have him dismissed from work. He says they are spreading malicious rumours about his sexuality and with the help of the CIA have bugged his office. In the first week of his admission he is observed to be responding to unseen stimuli when alone in his room. His family state that he is a lovely lad who never gets into any trouble with drink or drugs. They are very worried because in the last 3 months he has told them he can hear people talking about him to each other when he lies in bed at night. He has no significant medical history. Which one of the following courses of action would be most appropriate?

- ❏ A Commence chlorpromazine
- ❏ B Commence clozapine
- ❏ C Commence chlorpromazine with lorazepam and procyclidine as required
- ❏ D Commence olanzapine with lorazepam and procyclidine as required
- ❏ E Observe with sedation as required

Multiple Choice Questions

Mark your answers with a tick (True) or a cross (False) in the box provided. Leave the box blank for 'Don't know'. Do not look at the answers until you have completed the whole question paper.

2.16   Spastic paraparesis

❏   A   Means that an arm and a leg are affected by an upper motor neurone lesion
❏   B   In young women is most commonly caused by multiple sclerosis
❏   C   When caused by degenerative disc disease has a poor outcome
❏   D   Does not usually affect joint position sense
❏   E   Often produces bladder symptoms

2.17   Sacroiliitis occurs in

❏   A   Rheumatoid arthritis
❏   B   Ankylosing spondylitis
❏   C   Ulcerative colitis
❏   D   Reiter's syndrome
❏   E   Gout

2.18   Drug-induced diarrhoea is seen with

❏   A   Aluminium hydroxide
❏   B   Erythromycin
❏   C   Broad-spectrum antibiotics
❏   D   Imipramine
❏   E   Loperamide

2.19   The following are causes of clubbing

❏   A   Coeliac disease
❏   B   Atrial septal defect
❏   C   Cryptogenic fibrosing alveolitis
❏   D   Bronchiectasis
❏   E   COPD

2.20   Increased skin pigmentation occurs with

❏   A   Hypopituitarism
❏   B   Haemochromatosis
❏   C   Chronic renal failure
❏   D   Varicose eczema
❏   E   Vitiligo

2.21   Regarding hepatitis A infection

❏   A   10% of patients develop liver cirrhosis
❏   B   Anorexia is a prominent early symptom
❏   C   It may be spread by faecal contamination
❏   D   It may be fatal
❏   E   It always requires admission to an isolation unit

2.22   Severe acute abdominal pain is a feature of

❏   A   Coeliac disease
❏   B   Acute intermittent porphyria
❏   C   Lower lobe pneumonia
❏   D   Diabetic ketoacidosis
❏   E   Infection with herpes zoster at T10

2.23   Difficulty swallowing can occur as a result of the following conditions

❏   A   Oesophageal reflux
❏   B   Carcinoma of the stomach
❏   C   Motor neurone disease
❏   D   Depression
❏   E   Recurrent laryngeal nerve palsy

2.24   Regarding lung cancer

❏   A   Smokers tend to develop adenocarcinoma
❏   B   Vocal cord palsy indicates inoperability
❏   C   Tumours are more easily resected if close to the hilum
❏   D   Small-cell carcinoma can be treated by chemotherapy
❏   E   The brain is a common site for metastases

2.25   Proximal muscle weakness is a well recognised feature of

❏   A   Osteoporosis
❏   B   Thyrotoxicosis
❏   C   Corticosteroid therapy
❏   D   Muscular dystrophy
❏   E   Diabetes mellitus

2.26   The following are true of renal amyloid

❏   A   It produces large kidneys
❏   B   Prognosis is poor
❏   C   Staining with Congo red is characteristic
❏   D   It may present with chronic renal failure
❏   E   It may be caused by chronic infection

2.27   The following skin lesions are correctly paired with the disease stated

❏   A   Pyoderma gangrenosum – diabetes mellitus
❏   B   Erythema multiforme – rheumatic fever
❏   C   Rose spots – typhoid fever
❏   D   Skin ulcers – sickle cell anaemia
❏   E   Erythema nodosum – ulcerative colitis

2.28   Increased sweating is a recognised feature of

❏   A   Diabetic ketoacidosis
❏   B   Phaeochromocytoma
❏   C   Left ventricular failure
❏   D   Cystic fibrosis
❏   E   Acromegaly

2.29   Herpes simplex virus may

❏   A   Produce a severe generalised eruption in children with eczema
❏   B   Cause corneal lesions
❏   C   Cause encephalitis
❏   D   Be sensitive to aciclovir
❏   E   Result in post-herpetic neuralgia

2.30   Gynaecomastia is a feature of

☐ ʼ A   Lung cancer
☐ B   Old age
☐ C   Obesity
☐ D   Hypothyroidism
☐ E   Hypercholesterolaemia

2.31   An acute asthmatic attack may be precipitated by

☐ A   Exercise
☐ B   Selective beta-1 receptor-blocking drugs
☐ C   Prednisolone
☐ D   Ibuprofen
☐ E   Adrenaline

2.32   Causes of generalised lymphadenopathy include

☐ A   Sarcoid
☐ B   Lymphoma
☐ C   Tuberculosis
☐ D   Chronic lymphocytic lymphoma
☐ E   Lymphoedema

2.33   The following are causes of diastolic murmurs

☐ A   Austin Flint murmur
☐ B   Graham Steell murmur
☐ C   Mitral valve prolapse
☐ D   Mitral regurgitation
☐ E   Pulmonary regurgitation

2.34   Causes of a large tongue include

☐ A   Vitamin B_{12} deficiency
☐ B   Acromegaly
☐ C   Down's syndrome
☐ D   Amyloid
☐ E   Syphilis

2.35   Dementia

❏   A   Is termed presenile if it occurs before the age of 75
❏   B   Is always progressive
❏   C   May be caused by head injury
❏   D   Can be diagnosed by a mini mental test score of 6
❏   E   Causes a reversal of the sleep-wake cycle

2.36   The following refer to pulmonary tuberculosis

❏   A   It is unlikely if the chest X-ray is normal
❏   B   A Heaf test of >10 mm is suggestive
❏   C   *Mycobacterium* bacillus can be grown from blood culture
❏   D   The BCG vaccine is >90% protective for life
❏   E   Rifampicin causes optic neuropathy

2.37   Dark urine occurs with

❏   A   Beetroot consumption
❏   B   Heavy proteinuria
❏   C   Porphyria
❏   D   Malaria
❏   E   Gilbert's syndrome

2.38   Interferon may be of benefit in the following

❏   A   Hepatitis A
❏   B   Chronic hepatitis B
❏   C   Chronic hepatitis C
❏   D   Multiple sclerosis
❏   E   Depression

2.39   The following may provoke an epileptic seizure

❏   A   Flashing lights
❏   B   Illness
❏   C   Head injury
❏   D   Family argument
❏   E   Anticonvulsants

2.40 **The management of osteoporosis includes**

- ❏ A Avoiding exercise whenever possible
- ❏ B Stopping smoking
- ❏ C Increasing dietary calcium
- ❏ D Hormone replacement therapy
- ❏ E Avoiding travel by aeroplane

2.41 **The following drugs have been shown to decrease mortality after myocardial infarction**

- ❏ A Aspirin
- ❏ B Beta-blockers
- ❏ C rTPA
- ❏ D ACE inhibitors
- ❏ E Oral magnesium

2.42 **Hypothyroidism may cause**

- ❏ A Dementia
- ❏ B Hypothermia
- ❏ C Hirsutism
- ❏ D Coma
- ❏ E Pretibial myxoedema

2.43 **Ulceration inside the mouth occurs in**

- ❏ A Behçet's syndrome
- ❏ B Ulcerative colitis
- ❏ C SLE
- ❏ D Pemphigus vulgaris
- ❏ E Stress

2.44 **Risk factors for large bowel malignancy include**

- ❏ A Constipation
- ❏ B Family history
- ❏ C Ulcerative colitis
- ❏ D Crohn's disease
- ❏ E Diverticular disease

2.45   The following are features of a cerebellopontine angle tumour

- ❏ A   Facial weakness
- ❏ B   Facial numbness
- ❏ C   Deafness
- ❏ D   Ataxia
- ❏ E   Optic atrophy

2.46   The following suggest a median nerve injury

- ❏ A   Inability to oppose the thumb to the little finger
- ❏ B   Inability to adduct the thumb
- ❏ C   Sensory loss over the medial one and a half fingers
- ❏ D   Pain in the upper arm
- ❏ E   Tingling in the forearm

2.47   In elderly people

- ❏ A   A UTI may cause coma
- ❏ B   Part III accommodation is only for people who are continent
- ❏ C   Erythema ab igne may indicate hypothyroidism
- ❏ D   Cardiopulmonary resuscitation should not be performed on patients over the age of 85
- ❏ E   A haemoglobin level of 10 g/dl is within the normal range

2.48   Causes of an eosinophilia include

- ❏ A   Asthma
- ❏ B   Hodgkin's lymphoma
- ❏ C   Psoriasis
- ❏ D   Eczema
- ❏ E   Rheumatoid arthritis

2.49   A pleural effusion is often associated with

- ❏ A   Oesophageal rupture
- ❏ B   COPD
- ❏ C   Sarcoid
- ❏ D   Liver cirrhosis
- ❏ E   Diabetic ketoacidosis

2.50   Regarding left ventricular failure

- ❑   A   Frusemide is used acutely for its immediate diuretic effect
- ❑   B   ACE inhibitors decrease mortality and morbidity
- ❑   C   A change in heart size on chest radiograph will be visible within 24 h of treatment for the acute attack
- ❑   D   A gallop rhythm indicates inadequate treatment
- ❑   E   Pulsus alternans indicates a poor prognosis

2.51   The following can produce symptoms suggestive of schizophrenia

- ❑   A   Amphetamine addiction
- ❑   B   Pregnancy
- ❑   C   Opiate abuse
- ❑   D   Temporal lobe epilepsy
- ❑   E   Hypoglycaemia

2.52   Hirsutism is caused by

- ❑   A   Polycystic ovarian syndrome
- ❑   B   Congenital adrenal hyperplasia
- ❑   C   Porphyria cutanea tarda
- ❑   D   Acromegaly
- ❑   E   Thyrotoxicosis

2.53   Abnormal speech is a recognised feature of

- ❑   A   Ill-fitting dentures
- ❑   B   Parkinson's disease
- ❑   C   Motor neurone disease
- ❑   D   Multiple sclerosis
- ❑   E   Hypoglossal nerve damage

2.54   Ulcerative colitis is associated with

- ❑   A   Dermatitis herpetiformis
- ❑   B   Erythema nodosum
- ❑   C   Liver cirrhosis
- ❑   D   Arthritis
- ❑   E   Sclerosing cholangitis

2.55   The following refer to splitting of the second heart sound

☐   A   Reversed splitting occurs in left bundle branch block
☐   B   Fixed splitting occurs only in an atrial septal defect
☐   C   Wide splitting occurs in pulmonary stenosis
☐   D   It is normal to hear splitting in the mitral area
☐   E   The aortic second sound is louder in aortic stenosis

2.56   The following infectious diseases are transmitted by ticks

☐   A   Malaria
☐   B   Dengue fever
☐   C   Chagas disease
☐   D   Lyme disease
☐   E   Yellow fever

2.57   The following are true

☐   A   In a normal distribution, the mean, mode, and median may be but
        are not always the same
☐   B   The median is the most frequently occurring value
☐   C   The standard deviation refers to a measure of the spread of a
        normally distributed population
☐   D   In a normal distribution, ±1 SD includes 68% of the population
☐   E   In a normal distribution, ±3 SD includes 99% of the population

2.58   The following are true

☐   A   The standard error of the mean = the standard deviation divided
        by the square of the number of values in the sample
☐   B   A p value of 0.005 implies statistical significance
☐   C   A type 1 error results in a significant difference being obtained
        when it should not have been
☐   D   A paired t-test may be used for comparison of means for normally
        distributed populations only
☐   E   The chi-squared test may be performed on means

2.59   Photosensitivity occurs in

❑ A   SLE
❑ B   Amiodarone treatment
❑ C   Acute intermittent porphyria
❑ D   Pellagra
❑ E   Scurvy

2.60   Causes of chorea include

❑ A   Thyrotoxicosis
❑ B   Huntington's chorea
❑ C   Rheumatic fever
❑ D   Pregnancy
❑ E   Cerebellar lesion

——————————————— **END** ———————————————

**Go over your answers until your time is up. Correct answers
and teaching notes are overleaf**

BEST OF FIVE AND MULTIPLE CHOICE QUESTION PAPER 2
Answers

The correct answer options for each question are given below.

2.1	C	2.31	A B D
2.2	D	2.32	A B C D
2.3	B	2.33	A B E
2.4	D	2.34	B C D
2.5	D	2.35	C E
2.6	E	2.36	A E
2.7	A	2.37	A C D
2.8	A	2.38	B C D
2.9	E	2.39	A B C D E
2.10	E	2.40	B C D
2.11	E	2.41	A B C D
2.12	D	2.42	A B D
2.13	B	2.43	A D E
2.14	B	2.44	A B C
2.15	D	2.45	A B C D
2.16	B E	2.46	A E
2.17	B C D	2.47	A B C
2.18	B C	2.48	A B D E
2.19	A C D	2.49	A D
2.20	B C D	2.50	B C D E
2.21	B C D	2.51	A B C D E
2.22	B C D E	2.52	A B C D E
2.23	B C D	2.53	A B C D E
2.24	B D E	2.54	B C D E
2.25	B C D E	2.55	A B C
2.26	A B C D E	2.56	D
2.27	A C D E	2.57	C D E
2.28	B C E	2.58	B C D
2.29	A B C D	2.59	A B D
2.30	A B	2.60	A B C D

BEST OF FIVE AND MULTIPLE CHOICE QUESTION PAPER 2
Answers and Teaching Notes

2.1 C: Commence oral metronidazole

Clostridium difficile is a common problem within hospital medicine, frequently complicating the inpatient admission of elderly patients. It produces a necrotising toxin that may lead to the development of pseudomembranous colitis in severe cases. With the common prescribing of antibiotics, in particular third-generation cephalosporins and clindamycin, it should be suspected in all patients with diarrhoea following the commencement of antibiotics. Simple diarrhoea is of course a side-effect of antibiotics too, however the colour and distinct foul odour will often clinch the diagnosis before stool serology (for the toxin) confirms the diagnosis. Initial treatment is with oral metronidazole. Should this be unsuccessful second-line treatment is with oral vancomycin. Supportive therapy is also important but not sufficient in isolation.

2.2 D: Ultrasound scan of the abdomen

The LFTs demonstrate an obstructive picture. Abnormal LFTs may be divided into three broad categories – obstructive, hepatitic (parenchymal) and mixed. These reflect the underlying disease process and narrow the potential differential diagnoses. Although all of the tests listed could potentially be of value, with the exception of the PABA test, investigation should begin with an ultrasound of the abdomen. It is cheap, simple, non-invasive, readily available and will assist in guiding further investigation. It will demonstrate any intra- or extra-hepatic duct dilatation, liver size, shape and consistency along with the details of the gallbladder and pancreas. ERCP and CT abdomen may be requested following ultrasound. The PABA test is used in the diagnosis of pancreatic insufficiency.

2.3 B: *Staphylococcus aureus*

A red, hot swollen joint is one of the few rheumatological emergencies an undergraduate might be expected to know how to treat in depth. The differential diagnoses are wide – the commonest being gout/pseudogout and septic arthritis. It is paramount that septic arthritis is considered and treated urgently or treated until firmly excluded by joint aspiration. The joint aspirate itself may appear purulent and a raised white cell count (mostly neutrophils) will confirm the clinical suspicion. A joint may be destroyed within 24 h if left untreated. The consequences for a prosthetic joint may be even more profound. The commonest pathogen is *Staphylococcus aureus*. The empirical antibiotic regime of choice is flucloxacillin 6-hourly and fusidic acid 500 mg 8-hourly. Intravenous drugs should be used for 2 weeks and a total course of 6 weeks completed.

2.4 D: Demonstrates any metastatic disease not found at CT

Positron emission tomography (PET) imaging is a growing niche in nuclear medical imaging. It is most useful when combined with CT imaging – known as PET-CT. When used together it combines functional (nuclear) and structural (CT) imaging with impressive results. It has a growing, but in some areas not entirely confirmed, role in the management of cancer patients. Two arenas where it has shown greatest potential are in staging bronchial and oesophageal malignancies. By using the radionucleotide fluoro-deoxyglucose ([18]FDG) it can demonstrate glucose-avid areas indicative of increased metabolism. Tumours such as bronchial carcinoma are glucose-avid as the cancer cells have altered glucose metabolism. Therefore, both the primary tumour and any metastases will be highlighted. These may then be correlated with the findings on CT. Its value lies in identifying any areas of metastatic tissue not seen on conventional CT which may then exclude the patient from unnecessary surgical intervention.

2.5 D: Phosphate

This patient suffers from alcohol dependency and is suffering from alcohol withdrawal. This typically occurs from 12 h after the last consumption of alcohol. In scenarios such as this the cause may simply be lack of money to buy the volume of alcohol usually consumed. Poor personal hygiene and nutritional status is a reflection of how dominant alcohol is in the patient's life. With financial constraints, eating becomes secondary to alcohol in competing for available money. Therefore, these patients are commonly nutritionally depleted. It may first manifest itself following admission to hospital due to abstention from alcohol and access to nutritious meals.

Although a number of electrolyte imbalances may occur, including magnesium and potassium, it is the level of serum phosphate which one should be especially aware of and take precautions to monitor closely. Following the recommencement of feeding (re-feeding) levels may plummet dangerously low and require prompt replacement with intravenous phosphate. This is usually given as an intravenous infusion (IVI) of dipotassium hydrogen phosphate. A similar problem may occur with re-feeding for any reason – the re-feeding syndrome.

2.6 E: Spironolactone

This patient is an arteriopath with established heart failure. Heart failure is a hugely prevalent disease for which medications can be in the broadest sense divided into those with symptomatic benefit alone and those with prognostic benefits (but often help with symptoms too).

Prognostic benefit

Drug	Trials
Selective beta-blockers	CORERNICUS, MERIT-HF, ISIS
ACE inhibitors	SAVE, HOPE, CHARM
Angiotensin II antagonists	
Spironolactone (K-sparing diuretic)	RALES

Symptomatic benefit

Loop diuretics
Digoxin
Vasodilators (nitrates and hydralazine)

Heart transplant remains a limited option for certain specific patient groups.

2.7 A: pH: 7.27, PaO_2: 7.1, PCO_2: 8.9, HCO_3^-: 33.20, BE –4.9 mmol

Chronic obstructive pulmonary disease (COPD) is a very common disease requiring admission to hospital. Exacerbations may be infective or non-infective in nature. The spectrum of disease ranges from those with a relatively limited exercise tolerance to patients requiring home oxygen and nebulisers even to stay within the confines of their own home. Respiratory reserve is poor and susceptibility to infection is high. A lower respiratory tract infection (LRTI) can quickly lead to a dramatic deterioration in breathing which not infrequently warrants respiratory support in the form of non-invasive positive pressure ventilation (NIPPV) or HDU/ICU admission. Type II respiratory failure would commonly be the problem – both a low oxygen (HYPOXIC) and an elevated CO_2 (HYPERCAPNIA) is observed. Clinically hypercapnia may manifest as warm, dilated peripheries, with a flap (CO_2 retention asterixis) and papilloedema. An ABG in these patients typically shows a type II respiratory picture with an acidosis (low pH) and a degree of metabolic compensation giving rise to a raised bicarbonate (HCO_3^-).

2.8 A: Needle aspiration

The management of a pneumothorax is dependent on a number of factors. The patient described in this question is typical of those with underlying pleural blebs – inherent weaknesses in the pleural lining leading to recurrent spontaneous pneumothoraces. These patients are classically tall, thin, young men. All patients with pre-existing lung disease are more susceptible to sustaining a pneumothorax and for this reason this is one of the vital aspects to take into consideration when deciding the best course of action. Symptoms should also be factored in with the chosen course of treatment. Tension pneumothorax is rapidly fatal and requires immediate treatment with needle decompression and placement of a chest drain. This is likely to be a clinical rather than radiological diagnosis. A proportion of spontaneous pneumothoraces will also require a chest drain (see below). Those with recurrent pneumothorcaces (3 or more) should be considered for definitive surgical treatment – usually with pleurodesis.

Management of pneumothorax

Nature of pneumothorax	Treatment
<20%	Observe
>20%, <50%	Needle aspiration
>50%	Chest drain insertion
Recurrence	Pleurodesis/pleurectomy

2.9 E: Enrol in biological therapy programme

Rheumatoid disease (RD) should be treated with disease-modifying anti-rheumatic drugs (DMARDS) from diagnosis. It is an aggressive multisystem disease with joint pathology as its most frequent cause for presentation and relapse ('flare'). DMARDS may be supplemented with analgesic anti-inflammatory medications. A number of DMARDS are available with variable response, even with the same drug in different patients. Methotrexate is considered the first-line agent of choice.

DMARDS in rheumatoid disease

Methotrexate
Leflunomide
Sulphasalazine
Oral & im gold
Penicillamine
Hydroxychloroquine

This patient has highly active disease despite having tried three previous agents for a therapeutic treatment duration. In some circumstances dual DMARD therapy would be prescribed under specialist guidance, however this patient is a candidate for biological treatments. National Institute of Clinical Excellence (NICE) guidelines recommend the use of these agents (infliximab and etanercept) in adults with highly active rheumatic disease who have failed to respond to at least two standard DMARDS, including methotrexate. Biological therapies are cytokine inhibitors, with the early and still most commonly prescribed medications being those against tumour necrosis factor (TNF). In addition to etanercept and infliximab other therapies are being introduced including adalimumab. These drugs are largely administered by subcutaneous injections allowing patients, following appropriate education, to inject themselves in a similar manner to diabetics. Biological therapies inhibit the immune system, making patients more susceptible to infection and impairing wound healing. For a period before and after surgery these drugs must be discontinued.

2.10 E: PCO$_2$ 2.5 + HCO$_3^-$ 17.5

This patient has a profound metabolic acidosis. When a metabolic acidosis is identified two points should be considered further. Firstly is there a normal or abnormal anion gap? An abnormal anion gap (>12 mmol/l) suggests an exogenous source of acid; for example, lactate, as in this clinical scenario. Other examples would include an overdose of aspirin or ingestion of anti-freeze (ethane-1-2-diol).

Calculation of anion gap = $(Na^+ + K^+) - (HCO_3^- + Cl^-)$

Secondly, is there any degree of respiratory compensation – partial or complete? Complete implies the pH is correct to normal.

The source of exogenous acid in this case is clear – lactate has been recorded on the ABG analysis and is significantly elevated. The ischaemic leg, devoid of adequate oxygenation, is producing lactic acid from anaerobic metabolism within the muscles of the leg. The respiratory distress is the attempt at compensation of the acidosis – exhaling CO_2 through an increased respiratory rate. Remember $CO_2 + H_2O = H_2CO_3 = H^+(ACID) + HCO_3^-$. Likewise the HCO_3^- will be low due to the metabolic acidosis. The combination of PCO_2 2.5 + HCO_3^- 17.5 fits the bill.

2.11 E: Multi-infarct dementia

Dementia is a state of cognitive decline and disability. There is a global impairment of memory, personality and intellect without alteration of consciousness. The commonest type is Alzheimer's disease – an idiopathic state characterised by the presence of amyloid plaques and tau-protein neurofibrillary tangles within the brain. However, there are a number of other diseases which present with similar clinical features, albeit with some individual characteristics. One such feature is a stepwise deterioration in the cognitive status in multi-infarct (vascular) dementia, typically in those with pre-existing vascular disease (arteriopaths). This patient is a prime example with an extensive history of arterial disease and a relatively sudden deterioration noted by his daughter. Essentially, repeated small cerebrovascular accidents have taken place within the brain.

Types of dementia	Characteristic features
Pick's disease	Frontal lobe features
Alzheimer's disease	**After exclusion of other types**
Normal pressure hydrocephalus	Urinary incontinence and gait abnormalities
Sporadic CJD	Urinary incontinence and gait abnormalities
Multi-infarct dementia	Step wise fashion

Other more unusual forms of dementia include Huntingdon's disease, hypothyroidism and AIDS associated dementia.

Every attempt should be made at the time of presentation to identify a reversible cause for dementia.

2.12 D: Squamous cell bronchial carcinoma

A focal lung mass in a smoker should always be viewed with great suspicion, although there are many causes of focal lung lesions on CXR (see below).

Focal lung masses on CXR

- Bronchial carcinoma
- Abscess
- Encysted pleural effusion
- Nipple(s)
- Hamartoma
- Tuberculosis
- Infarction
- Granulomas
- Pulmonary metastasis
- Rheumatoid nodule

Bronchial carcinoma is divided histologically into small (oat) cell and non-small-cell types. Non-small-cell is further divided into at least three subtypes (see below).

Types of bronchial carcinoma
- *Small cell*
- *Non-small cell*
  Squamous cell
  Adenocarcinoma
  Alveolar cell
  Large cell

Differentiation is achieved following sampling of the tumorous tissue which typically is gained at bronchoscopy or image-guided biopsy. However, other features of a patient's history may indicate a suspicion of which subtype has occurred. Small-cell malignancies, being derived from the APUD (endocrine) cells, are classically associated with paraneoplastic phenomena such as ectopic adrenocorticotrophic hormone (ACTH) (Cushing's syndrome) and the syndrome of inappropriate ADH (SIADH). In this case there is an elevated calcium level, which is a true rise given the normal albumin. Although hypercalcaemia is seen with bony metastatic disease (usually later in the disease course), this finding is typically seen in those with squamous cell bronchial carcinoma. It produces parathyroid-like hormone, stimulating the release of calcium by mimicking parathyroid hormone's action on bone, kidneys and the gut. On the clinical symptoms alone (haemoptysis, shortness or breath and weight loss) all the stems are feasible causes.

2.13 B: Right optic tract

An understanding of the main structures of the optic pathway will enable all visual defects to be localised.

The optic nerve carries nerve fibres from the retina to the optic chiasm.

The medial fibres (the lateral visual field) cross (decussate) the midline. The lateral fibres continue on the ipsilateral side with the fibres which have joined from the contralateral side to form the optic tracts.

The optic fibres run in the optic tract to the lateral geniculate nucleus. From here they continue in the optic radiations to the visual centre in the occipital lobe.

Visual field defects

Defect	Location in optic pathway
Complete loss one eye	Ipsilateral optic nerve
Bitemporal hemianopia	Optic chiasm
Right homonymous hemianopia	Left optic tract/radiation
Left homonymous hemianopia	Right optic tract/radiation

2.14 B: Exercise desaturation

Pneumocystis carinii pneumonia (PCP) is caused by the ubiquitous eukaryote *P. carinii*. It is an unusual condition in the normal population but a very real issue for the immunocompromised, in particular patients with acquired immunodeficiency syndrome (AIDS). Others at risk include individuals with haematological malignancies, organ transplant recipients and those receiving long-term steroid or cytotoxic therapy.

Plain CXR most often shows diffuse interstitial opacification, but can be entirely normal. Rarely pulmonary nodules that cavitate can be observed. High-resolution computed tomography (HRCT) is the imaging modality of choice.

The classical feature of PCP is desaturation on exercise. This may be demonstrated at ward level by measuring pulse oximetry both before and after walking up and down the ward and recording if a significant drop is observed.

2.15 D: Commence olanzapine with lorazepam and procyclidine as required

This man meets the diagnostic criteria for schizophrenia and should be started on antipsychotic medication. Best practice would be to commence an atypical antipsychotic. Atypical antipsychotics carry a lower risk of extrapyramidal side-effects. However, this risk is not removed completely, so it is appropriate to prescribe anticholinergic medication, such as procyclidine. The antipsychotic action of olanzapine cannot be expected to begin for at least 10 days. In the meantime its sedative action may be beneficial, but further sedation may be required. In these circumstances it is appropriate to prescribe a short-acting benzodiazepine such as lorazepam. Clozapine is the most effective medication for treatment-resistant schizophrenia, but carries a small risk of serious complications (see below) and so is usually reserved for patients for whom two antipsychotics given at an appropriate dose for 6–8 weeks have proved to be ineffective.

Serious adverse effects of clozapine

- Fatal agranulocytosis (1 in 5000)
- Fatal myocarditis or cardiomyopathy (1 in 1300)
- Fatal pulmonary embolus (1 in 4500)

Despite these adverse effects, clozapine reduces overall mortality in schizophrenia, largely because of a considerable reduction in the incidence of suicide.

2.16 Spastic paraparesis   Answers: B E

Spastic paraparesis refers to the upper motor neurone weakness of both legs.

In young women, demyelination (for example, multiple sclerosis) is the most likely cause but other important causes include:

- Cord compression – this needs to be above the level of L1: the cord ends here and lesions below it will not produce a spastic paraparesis. Causes include degenerative disc disease, disc prolapse and tumours. Degenerative disc disease/disc prolapse is amenable to surgery and usually produces excellent results: recovery may be full
- Motor neurone disease
- Birth injury
- Sub-acute combined degeneration of the cord
- Syringomyelia
- Para-sagittal meningioma

- Treponemal disease, generalised paralysis of the insane (GPI), taboparesis
- Hereditary, for example, Friedreich's ataxia.

Option D is difficult. Usually a spastic paraparesis will produce sensory and motor changes and joint position sense is often lost. There is an exception – motor neurone disease only affects motor neurones, therefore technically joint position sense is preserved.

Remember that in multiple sclerosis only the central nervous system is affected but both the motor and sensory systems can be involved. In motor neurone disease only the motor system is affected but both the central and peripheral nervous systems are involved.

2.17 Sacroiliitis   Answers: B C D
The easiest way to remember the causes of sacroiliitis is to think of the associations and causes of the seronegative spondarthritis: **PUB CAR**

Psoriasis
Ulcerative colitis
Behçet's disease
Crohn's disease
Ankylosing spondylitis
Reiter's disease

Note that Whipple's disease is seronegative but does not usually cause sacroiliitis.

2.18 Drug-induced diarrhoea   Answers: B C
Increased transit time (producing constipation) is caused by:

- Sympathetic nervous system stimulation
- Opiate receptor stimulation, for example codeine, loperamide
- Parasympathetic nervous system inhibition, for example anticholinergics and antidepressants
- Aluminium salts.

Decreased transit time (producing diarrhoea) is caused by:

- Parasympathetic nervous system stimulation
- Sympathetic nervous system inhibition
- Alteration of bacterial flora, for example antibiotic-associated diarrhoea or pseudomembranous colitis. Note that erythromycin also has a pro-kinetic effect on the gut as well as altering bacterial flora
- Magnesium salts.

2.19 Clubbing   Answers: A C D

Nail clubbing only occurs when fibrosis, infective or inflammatory conditions are chronic:

Heart
- Cyanotic congenital heart disease (atrial septal defect is not cyanotic)
- Subacute bacterial endocarditis

Lungs
- Infective or inflammatory: tuberculosis, bronchiectasis, lung abscess, empyema, bronchial carcinoma, mesothelioma
- Fibrotic: cryptogenic fibrosing alveolitis
- Chronic obstructive airways disease (COAD) is NOT a cause of clubbing – if it is present think of a co-existing malignancy

Gastrointestinal
- Inflammatory bowel disease, liver cirrhosis, coeliac disease, gastrointestinal lymphoma.

2.20 Skin pigmentation   Answers: B C D

Increased skin pigmentation has many causes:

- Raised melanin – haemochromatosis; Addison's disease – stimulates increased melanocyte-stimulating hormone (MSH) and ACTH; hyperthyroidism; renal failure – increased MSH-like hormone production
- Haemosiderin – extravasated blood from venous ulcers can cause localised melanin production
- Increased ACTH – ACTH also has MSH activity; Addison's disease; oat cell tumours of the bronchus; Cushing's disease.

Other causes of increased local pigmentation are:

- acanthosis nigricans
- systemic sclerosis
- pregnancy/oral contraceptive pill (OCP)
- neurofibromatosis.

2.21 Hepatitis A infection   Answers: B C D

Hepatitis A virus is spread by the faeco-oral route. It has an incubation period of about 2 weeks. The pre-icteric period is up to 2 weeks. During this time, patients experience nausea, vomiting, anorexia, headache and malaise. During the icteric period the patient often feels better. On examination, 10% have hepatomegaly; there may also be lymphadenopathy and in some cases a rash. Rarely, fulminant hepatitis develops resulting in coma and death.

Cirrhosis does not occur. Mild cases may be managed at home.

2.22 Acute abdominal pain   Answers: B C D E

Obvious causes of severe acute abdominal pain include infection, inflammation and perforation of abdominal organs.

Important causes include lower lobe pneumonia (the pain of which may be referred down as far as the right iliac fossa, mimicking appendicitis); diabetic ketoacidosis causing gastric stasis and ileus; thoracic *Herpes zoster*; acute intermittent porphyria.

Coeliac disease can cause abdominal distension or bloating but tends not to produce severe acute abdominal pain.

2.23 Dysphagia   Answers: B C D

See also Paper 1, Question 1.28. Oesophageal reflux tends to produce heartburn and retrosternal pain. Unless stricture formation has occurred dysphagia is not a usual feature.

Carcinoma of the stomach, in particular of the fundus, can compress the oesophagus, producing dysphagia.

Motor neurone disease causes weakness of the pharyngeal muscles.

Depression causes a functional dysphagia.

Recurrent laryngeal nerve palsy causes dysphasia, not dysphagia.

2.24 Lung cancer   Answers: B D E

Lung carcinoma is divided into small-cell and non-small-cell carcinoma:

- Small-cell carcinoma
  Oat cell – this arises from endocrine cells which secrete polypeptide hormones. These are highly malignant and rapid growing but respond well to chemotherapy.
- Non-small-cell carcinoma
  Squamous cell carcinoma – 40% of all lung carcinomas. Cavitates, metastasises late.
  Large-cell carcinomas – 25% of tumours; metastasises early.
  Adenocarcinoma – 10% of tumours. Arises in scar tissue, therefore is associated with asbestosis. Proportionally more common in non-smokers, women and elderly people.

Alveolar cell carcinoma – 1–2% of tumours. These patients produce large amounts of mucoid sputum.

The treatment for small-cell carcinoma is chemotherapy. For non-small-cell carcinoma the treatment is surgery with or without chemotherapy. Surgery is only an option if:

- the tumour is not too near the hilum
- there is no evidence of metastasis
- FEV_1 >1.5 l
- there is no vocal cord paralysis.

Carcinoma of the lung metastasises to brain, bone and liver.

2.25 Proximal muscle weakness   Answers: B C D E

Proximal muscle weakness means weakness predominantly affecting the shoulder/pelvic girdle. It is caused by:

- muscle disorders – for example, polymyositis, muscular dystrophy, myotonic dystrophy
- endocrine disorders – thyrotoxicosis, hypothyroidism, Cushing's disease
- metabolic disorders – osteomalacia, steroid therapy, hypokalaemia.

2.26 Renal amyloid   Answers: A B C D E

Small kidneys are usually a feature of most chronic renal disorders, the exceptions being hydronephrosis, polycystic renal disease and renal amyloid that produce large kidneys.

Amyloidosis is a disorder of protein metabolism. It consists of protein fibrils that stain red with Congo red and show a green fluorescence in polarised light. It may be primary or secondary to chronic infection. In the secondary form serum amyloid A, which is an acute phase protein, is overproduced and becomes deposited in organs.

2.27 Skin lesions   Answers: A C D E

Diabetes mellitus is associated with pyoderma gangrenosum and necrobiosis lipoidica. It may cause lipoatrophy or lipohypertrophy (related to insulin injection site), and certain skin infections (eg candidiasis) are more common in diabetics.

A previous stem referred to necrolytic migrating erythema; this is associated with a glucagonoma which can produce diabetes mellitus.

Rheumatic fever can cause erythema marginatum. Erythema multiforme is associated with herpes simplex infection (type 1), *Mycoplasma pneumoniae*, drugs such as sulphonamides and barbiturates, *Streptococcus*, *Yersinia* and neoplasia. In 50% of cases no cause is found. Rose spots are a macular papular rash appearing on the upper abdomen/thorax during the second week of a typhoid illness.

For causes of erythema nodosum see Paper 1, Question 1.17.

2.28 Sweating Answers: B C E

An increase in sympathetic nervous system activity occurs with anxiety, heart failure, phaeochromocytoma and fever.

In ketoacidosis there is profound dehydration and the skin is usually dry. Excess growth hormone affects the sweat glands, causing increased sweating and greasy skin.

The trick in this question is cystic fibrosis. Everyone remembers the abnormal sweat test and therefore marks this as true, but in fact it is the amount of sodium and not the amount of sweat that is increased.

2.29 Herpes simplex virus Answers: A B C D

Herpes simplex is a DNA pox virus. Type 1 causes oral lesions and type 2 causes genital lesions, but this is not absolute.

Trauma to the skin or a mucosal surface – for example, the eye, genital area or mouth – allows introduction of the virus. Primary infection of genital herpes is usually more severe than primary oral infection. The latter may be asymptomatic, or may cause marked localised pain, ulceration and systemic illness.

The virus lies dormant in the dorsal root ganglion and may periodically reactivate. In genital herpes, recurrences are inevitable.

People at risk of severe infection include:

- immunocompromised inpatients
- neonates (Caesarean section should be performed)
- atopic individuals (even if eczema is not in an active phase, eczema herpeticum may occur.

Post-herpetic neuralgia refers to the pain in the dermatome affected by shingles (Herpes zoster and not Herpes simplex).

2.30 Gynaecomastia   **Answers: A B**

Causes of gynaecomastia include:

- physiological – neonatal, puberty, old age
- endocrine – hyperthyroidism
- metabolic – starvation and refeeding, oestrogen excess and testosterone deficiency
- tumours – lung and testicular tumours producing human chorionic gonadotropin (hCG). Note therefore that testicular tumours can produce gynaecomastia by production of oestrogen or hCG
- drugs – see Paper 4, Question 4.30.

Obesity causes an increase in breast size due to fat deposition, but not true breast tissue development.

2.31 Acute asthma   **Answers: A B D**

Bronchial hyper-responsiveness is thought to be responsible for symptoms in asthma. The airways are thought to be more sensitive to cold air and irritants, such as dust. The immediate effect of exercise is bronchodilation followed by bronchoconstriction, the latter being exaggerated in asthmatic patients. Patients often complain that they are extremely short of breath 10–15 min after stopping exercise.

Airway tone is normally under the influence of the following:

- Sympathetic nerve system which dilates the airways via beta-2 receptor stimulation
- Parasympathetic nerve stimulation by the vagus nerve which induces bronchial constriction
- Cyclic AMP activation
- Numerous other receptors, for example adenosine receptors.

Although it is obvious that beta-2 receptor-blocking drugs will cause bronchial constriction, it must also be appreciated that even highly selective beta-1 receptor-blocking drugs have the potential to cause a fatal asthmatic attack and are contraindicated.

Drugs potentiating the sympathetic nervous system, such as adrenaline, will cause bronchial dilation and until quite recently adrenaline was first-line treatment for an asthmatic attack. Newer treatments include beta-2 receptor stimulation by drugs such as salbutamol and the longer acting salmeterol.

Drugs inhibiting the parasympathetic nervous system include ipratropium bromide which by its anticholinergic effect helps to relax the airways. The theophylline group of drugs are phosphodiesterase inhibitors which help to potentiate the effect of cyclic AMP and this also results in airway dilatation.

Bronchoconstriction is not the only problem during an acute asthmatic attack; in addition there is marked inflammation and steroids, such as prednisolone, have considerable benefit but take several hours to work.

However, drugs such as non-steroidal anti-inflammatories (NSAIDs) act by diverting the precursors from the cyclooxygenase to the lipoxygenase pathway, resulting in increased production of leukotrienes which are potent bronchoconstrictors. These drugs should therefore be avoided.

This is a very important question and frequently comes up.

2.32 Generalised lymphadenopathy　　　　　　Answers: A B C D

The causes of generalised lymphadenopathy are:

- lymphoma – lymph nodes are said to be rubbery and firm
- leukaemia – chronic lymphocytic leukaemia and acute lymphoblastic leukaemia in particular
- malignancies – the nodes tend to be very firm and asymmetrical
- infection: viral (eg CMV, HIV, infection, infectious mononucleosis); bacterial (eg TB, brucellosis); protozoan (eg toxoplasmosis)
- connective tissue diseases (eg rheumatoid arthritis, SLE)
- infiltrative/granulomatous disorders (eg sarcoid drugs, such as phenytoin).

Lymphoedema is caused by obstruction to lymphatic flow and does not produce a generalised lymphadenopathy.

2.33 Diastolic murmurs　　　　　　Answers: A B E

Diastolic murmurs may be divided into mid-diastolic or early diastolic. Mid-diastolic murmurs include the murmur of mitral stenosis, best heard at the apex with the patient on the left side, and accentuated on exertion. It is of low frequency and rumbling in nature.

Tricuspid stenosis is also mid-diastolic, best heard at the left sternal edge and louder on inspiration.

The Austin Flint murmur is produced when aortic regurgitation causes a jet of blood to hit the mitral valve; it is best heard at the apex.

Early diastolic murmurs – aortic regurgitation is best heard at the left sternal edge and the apex, with the patient sitting forward in held expiration. It is a blowing high-pitched murmur.

Pulmonary regurgitation is best heard on the right of the sternum, in held inspiration. It has a blowing sound and variable pitch.

The Graham Steell murmur is due to mitral stenosis causing pulmonary hypertension leading to pulmonary hypertension. It is best heard at the left sternal edge.

Systolic murmurs may be divided into ejection systolic, mid-systolic, pansystolic or late systolic.

- Ejection systolic murmurs include: aortic stenosis, pulmonary stenosis, atrial septal defects, hypertrophic cardiomyopathy, Fallot's tetralogy and flow murmurs (from aortic regurgitation or pulmonary regurgitation).
- Pansystolic murmurs include: mitral regurgitation – best heard at the apex to the axilla, flowing in nature; tricuspid regurgitation – best heard at the left sternal edge and low-pitched; ventricular septal defect – heard at the left sternal edge, loud and rough.
- Late systolic murmurs include: hypertrophic obstructive cardiac myopathy (note this may also produce an ejection mid-systolic murmur) – this murmur is best heard on standing; mitral valve prolapse – best heard at the apex; coarctation of the aorta – heard at the left sternal edge radiating to the back.

2.34 Large tongue
Answers: B C D

Amyloid of the AL type causes infiltration and hence enlargement of the tongue.

Acromegaly causes enlargement because of overgrowth of soft tissues. In Down's syndrome the tongue is said to be fissured and prominent (this may be relative to the size of the mouth rather than a true increase in size). Vitamin B_{12} deficiency causes a painful red tongue, but it is not enlarged.

2.35 Dementia
Answers: C E

Dementia is a decline in cognitive function in a setting of clear consciousness. It is usually but not always progressive and with treatment may even be improved.

It is termed pre-senile if it occurs before the age of 60. There is an hereditary pre-disposition to certain dementias and some (eg Pick's and Huntington's diseases) have a clear genetic basis.

Environmental agents, such as aluminium, prions and viruses, have also been implicated. Metabolic disorders such as hypothyroidism, vitamin B$_{12}$ deficiency, infection (eg neurosyphilis), head injury and cerebrovascular disease (eg multiple infarcts) may all cause dementia. It is thus essential to screen for these conditions and commence treatment to prevent further deterioration.

One of the early features of dementia, particularly of the Alzheimer's type, is a reversal of the sleep-wake cycle and patients are seen to wander at night. The mini mental test score is very helpful, but dementia should not be diagnosed from a single test. A score <6 should alert the clinician but dementia must be diagnosed on repeated assessments of the patient, interviews with the relatives and after exclusion of the conditions mentioned above.

2.36 Pulmonary tuberculosis   Answers: A E

Questions on pulmonary TB are extremely common in finals exams.
In the late 1980s the World Health Organisation (WHO) declared the rise in incidence of TB to be a global emergency.

Human tuberculosis is caused by infection with *Mycobacterium tuberculosis, M. bovis* or *M. africanum*.

Seventy-five per cent of new cases of TB involve the respiratory system. Pulmonary TB may produce a variety of abnormalities on chest X-ray, including cavitating lesions, hilar enlargement, nodules and consolidation. If the chest X-ray is normal, pulmonary TB is highly unlikely. (TB bronchitis may occur with a normal chest X-ray, but this is extremely rare.)

The diagnosis is made from the history, examination and clinical investigations. Blood cultures are not helpful as the *Mycobacterium* bacillus cannot be grown from blood. Acid-fast bacilli (AFB) can be obtained from sputum smears and gastric washings and conventionally it takes 6 weeks for the AFB to grow and drug sensitivities to be obtained. However, newer techniques involving the polymerase chain reaction (PCR) enable the diagnosis to be made more quickly. This is proving to be useful in cases of tuberculosis meningitis where PCR techniques can be applied to cerebrospinal fluid (CSF) samples.

Early morning urine specimens are used to look for renal TB.

Skin testing with the Mantoux or Heaf test may be useful. The Mantoux test involves purified peptide derivative (PPD) preparation being injected intra-dermally, a result being read 48–72 h later. The Heaf test involves placing PPD on to the skin and then piercing this area of skin with the six needles of the Heaf gun. The results of the tests are not always conclusive – in over-whelming TB the skin tests may be negative and routine immunisation of many individuals will lead them to have positive results anyway.

However, the Heaf and Mantoux tests are of use in determining which patients should be vaccinated. In general, if the standard concentration of PPD (100 unit/ml) is used then Heaf grades 0 and 1 or a Mantoux response of 0–4 mm indicates a negative response and patients may be offered the BCG immunisation in the absence of contraindications. Those with a grade 2 Heaf or a Mantoux reaction of 5–14 mm are considered positive and should not be vaccinated. Non-vaccinated individuals with a Heaf grade 3 or 4 or a Mantoux response >15 mm should be referred for specialist advice and consideration of prophylactic chemotherapy. The BCG vaccination is about 70–75% protective for about 20–30 years.

The treatment for pulmonary TB is frequently reviewed, but at the time of writing involves a 6-month regime. The initial phase lasts for 2 months and consists of daily rifampicin, isoniazid, pyrazinamide and ethambutol. The continuation phase lasts for a further 4 months and consists of daily rifampicin and isoniazid. Ethambutol may be omitted from the initial phase if there is a low risk of resistance to isoniazid.

Isoniazid may cause a peripheral neuropathy and it is customary to prescribe daily pyridoxine to prevent this. Ethambutol used to be a standard treatment, but it causes optic neuritis and is not now routinely used. The main side-effect of rifampicin is to alter liver enzymes and if bilirubin becomes elevated rifampicin should be stopped.

2.37 Dark urine   Answers: A C D

Dark urine may occur due to:

- pigments (eg beetroot)
- drugs (eg rifampicin)
- haemoglobin and its metabolic products (eg bilirubin)
- porphyria (urine darkens on standing)
- intravascular haemolysis (eg malaria – hence the term 'black water fever').

Conjugated bilirubin is water-soluble and appears in the urine but unconju-gated urine is colourless. Gilbert's syndrome is an hereditary condition where there is a lack of the conjugating enzyme producing increased unconjugated bilirubin.

Heavy proteinuria can cause the urine to be white and frothy.

2.38 Interferon   Answers: B C D

The two main forms of interferon used for treatment are alpha and beta interferon. Alpha interferon tends to boost the immune system and is therefore used to aid clearance of chronic viral infections, such as chronic hepatitis B and C. Beta interferon reduces immune-mediated destruction of tissue and has been used in trials in multiple sclerosis. However, its use is controversial: there is a minor reduction in length of stay in hospital for relapses but no reduction in mortality has been demonstrated. The drug is extremely expensive and should only be prescribed by a consultant neurologist.

The side-effects of both types of interferon include flu-like symptoms, myalgia and depression. Hepatitis A does not exist in a chronic state.

2.39 Epilepsy   Answers: A B C D E

It is well known that flashing lights can provoke a seizure. Illness, particularly causing a high fever, may precipitate fits especially in children. Head injury, cerebral infarction and brain tumours are causes of new-onset seizures. Anti-convulsant overdose produces cerebellar signs and can increase fit frequency. 'A family argument' is a question that has been reported by many candidates. The answer is true and the explanation is probably that it is due to stress, another well-recognised factor.

2.40 Osteoporosis   Answers: B C D

Management of osteoporosis includes prevention and treatment.

- Prevention: regular exercise throughout life; adequate dietary calcium; HRT when appropriate; moderate alcohol intake and stopping smoking.
- Treatment: general (ie pain relief, physiotherapy); specific (ie drugs to stimulate bone formation, eg fluoride); drugs to prevent bone resorption (eg HRT) – cyclical disodium etidronate with calcium carbonate, calcitonin and calcium.

All patients should receive supplemental calcium and where an additional anti-resorptive agent is indicated the initial choice is between a bisphosphonate (eg etidronate) and HRT.

2.41 Post-myocardial infarction   Answers: A B C D

Although there have been many trials looking at mortality after myocardial infarction, the most important ones to know about are the ISIS (International Study of Infarct Survival) trials.

ISIS I examined the effect of beta-blockade within 12 h of the onset of chest pain. The result showed a reduction in mortality of 15% at 7 days. The mechanism was thought to be prevention of cardiac rupture, reduction of arrhythmia and limitation of infarct size.

ISIS II measured the 5-week mortality. Patients were randomised into four groups:

- 1.5 million units of streptokinase – 25% reduction in mortality
- Aspirin – 23% reduction in mortality
- Streptokinase plus aspirin – 42% reduction in mortality
- Placebo.

The importance of ISIS II was that the effects of streptokinase and aspirin were additive.

ISIS III looked at different thrombolytic agents. It was found that there was no significant advantage with the newer, more expensive agents and streptokinase was therefore the first-line treatment. However, subsequent studies, including GISSI II and GUSTO, showed the benefit of recombinant tissue plasminogen activator (rTPA).

rTPA should be given to patients who are eligible for thrombolytic therapy who

- have an anterior MI and are under 65 years
- have a known allergy to streptokinase
- have a recent (<1 month) proven streptococcal infection
- have had streptokinase >5 days ago and <1 year ago.

Note that policies differ between hospitals.

ISIS IV examined the effects of ACE inhibition after myocardial infarction. A further 7% reduction in mortality was noted at 5 weeks. Numerous other studies have confirmed the beneficial effect of ACE inhibition. It is now common practice to give ACE inhibitors to patients with clinical evidence of heart failure or impaired LV function (eg demonstrated by echocardiography) or who have extensive Q wave infarction.

The role of magnesium is controversial. Some studies supported the use of magnesium, others did not. The question refers to oral magnesium which has not been shown to be of benefit.

2.42 Hypothyroidism   Answers: A B D

Hypothyroidism is an important endocrine condition with widespread effects on the body.

- Skin (often dry, peripherally cyanosed, cold and swollen; peri-orbital oedema, xanthelasma and associated autoimmune conditions, eg vitiligo)
- Cardiovascular system (bradycardia, low volume pulse, pericardial effusion)
- Respiratory system (pleural effusion)
- Central nervous system (speech – this may be slow or hoarse; hearing – nerve deafness which may be bilateral; cognitive function – depression/dementia)
- Peripheral nervous system (proximal myopathy, delayed relaxation of reflex jerks; carpal tunnel syndrome)
- Anaemia (macrocytic – associated with pernicious anaemia; microcytic – iron deficiency, for example, due to menorrhagia)
- Hypercholesterolaemia
- Hypothermia.

In the severe form a patient may present in coma and careful thyroxine replacement is necessary.

Hirsutism is not a feature. In fact, loss of hair occurs.

Pre-tibial myxoedema is an unfortunate term because 'myxoedema' is another term for hypothyroidism but in fact this condition occurs in hyper-thyroidism.

2.43 Mouth ulceration   Answers: A D E

It is worth learning a list of diseases that cause ulceration inside the mouth and diseases that cause genital ulceration as questions are often asked about these.

Causes of oral and/or genital ulceration:

- Behçet's disease
- Reiter's disease
- Crohn's disease
- Strachan's syndrome

- Herpes simplex, types 1 and 2
- Syphilis
- Pemphigus.

Ulcerative colitis does not cause oral or genital ulceration, whereas Crohn's disease can cause both. Stress can cause aphthous mouth ulcers but not genital ulcers.

2.44 Colonic carcinoma   Answers: A B C

Familial adenomatous polyposis accounts for 1% of all cases of carcinoma of the colon. (See Paper 4, Question 4.28)

Hereditary non-polyposis colon cancer is an autosomal dominant condition, the gene of which has been localised to chromosome 2. It accounts for 5–15% of cases of carcinoma of the colon. A few adenomatous polyps develop which rapidly transform to cancer.

Ulcerative colitis predisposes to malignancy (after 10 years of colitis, malignant foci in the large bowel are frequent). Crohn's disease is associated with a slight increase in colonic carcinoma, but this is not as common as in ulcerative colitis.

Recent evidence has suggested that constipation allows increased time for carcinogens to lie in contact with the bowel wall, predisposing to malignancy.

Diverticular disease itself does not predispose to malignancy.

2.45 Cerebellopontine angle lesions   Answers: A B C D

The key to this question is knowledge of the neuroanatomy. In the cerebellopontine angle are the cerebellar tracts, the Vth, VIIth and VIIIth cranial nerves. From this it can be deduced that tumours in this area may cause facial numbness (damage to V), weakness (damage to VII), deafness (damage to VIII) and ataxia (cerebellar pathway damage).

2.46 Median nerve   Answers: A E

The median nerve supplies the muscles of the hand which may be remembered by use of the mnemonic **LOAF**:

Lumbricals I & II
Opponens pollicis
Abductor pollicis
Flexor pollicis brevis

The ulnar nerve supplies the rest of the muscles of the hand, including adduction of the thumb.

Sensation: the lateral 3½ fingers are supplied by the median nerve; the ulnar nerve supplies the medial 1½ fingers.

Tingling in the arm is a common symptom of carpal tunnel syndrome (as is pain in the forearm) but pain in the upper arm is not.

2.47 Care of the elderly   Answers: A B C

Altered behaviour/confusion is a common presenting symptom of infection in the elderly; even a urinary tract infection (UTI) may cause symptoms suggestive of a dementia or even produce a coma. The elderly are more prone to hypothyroidism and sensitivity to the cold encourages them to sit close to fires, producing erythema ab igne.

Part III accommodation is only for people who are continent; incontinent people need to be considered for nursing homes.

A haemoglobin of 10 g/dl is not within the normal range – it is too low. Cardiopulmonary resuscitation should not be performed on the basis of age.

2.48 Eosinophilia   Answer: A B D E

The normal eosinophil count is (0.04–0.4) ×10⁹/l and may be raised 100- or even 1000-fold in disease states. Causes of eosinophilia include:

- infection – fungi, parasites
- drugs (eg sulphonamides, tetracyclines, nitrofurantoin, NSAIDs)
- vasculitis (eg Churg–Strauss syndrome, which is defined as asthma, eosinophilia and vasculitis affecting two or more organs apart from the lungs); but any other cause of a vasculitis may cause eosinophilia – eg rheumatoid arthritis
- dermatological conditions (eg eczema, scabies, pemphigus, pemphigoid)
- malignancy – lymphoproliferative disease, such as Hodgkin's disease; myeloproliferative disease such as hypereosinophilic syndrome.

2.49 Pleural effusion   Answers: A D

Oesophageal rupture causes leakage of fluid into the mediastinum and a pleural effusion is common. Liver cirrhosis causes a pleural effusion due to hypo-albuminaemia and the effusion is therefore a transudate. Sarcoid rarely produces a pleural effusion; more commonly it produces reticular nodular shadowing with hilar enlargement and fibrosis.

COPD does not produce a pleural effusion and its presence may be indicative of coexisting heart failure or an underlying malignancy.

Diabetic ketoacidosis does not produce a pleural effusion. In the initial stage the patient is hypovolaemic, but if fluid replacement is excessive then heart failure and pleural effusions may develop.

2.50 Left ventricular failure   Answers: B C D E

Acute left ventricular failure (LVF) is one of the most important medical emergencies. The patient must be assessed with regard to ABC (ie airway, breathing and circulation). If the airway is patent and breathing is adequate, attention needs to be paid to circulation. Intravenous access by use of a large-bore cannula must be obtained. The patient needs to be sitting upright breathing 100% oxygen (unless there is a clear history of COAD). Management depends on the state of the patient; for example, if moribund, hypotensive and unable to breathe then ventilation may be appropriate. However, if the patient is well enough, information may be obtained to confirm a history of LVF, ie orthopnoea, paroxysmal nocturnal dyspnoea and precipitating factors, such as MI, change of medication or arrhythmia may become apparent.

Examination: the clinical features of LVF include tachycardia with a weak, low-volume pulse; a low systolic blood pressure; a displaced apex beat (displaced laterally and inferiorly) and on auscultation a third heart sound may be heard, producing a gallop rhythm. When the heartbeat alternates between good and then poor volume (pulsus alternans) the heart failure is severe and indicates a poor prognosis.

Basic investigations: FBC, U&Es, cardiac enzymes if appropriate, ECG, chest radiograph, temperature and urinalysis.

Drug treatment includes oxygen at the highest concentration tolerated; IV diamorphine (plus anti-emetic). Diamorphine dilates pulmonary veins and therefore reduces the work of the heart and it also relieves the sensation of breathlessness. IV frusemide has a rapid venodilator action in the lungs; its diuretic action takes time to have an effect.

Angiotensin converting enzyme (ACE) inhibitors decrease mortality and morbidity in LVF.

It is worth remembering the pathophysiology of LVF. The heart is a muscular pump. As it fails the heart gets bigger and pumps less efficiently. A back pressure develops and the pulmonary venous pressure rises. As it rises further fluid is squeezed out of the veins into the lung interstitium and can be seen as septal lines (Kerley B lines) and fluid in the horizontal fissure. As the pressure rises further fluid accumulates in the alveoli, giving the typical 'fluffy' shadowing on chest radiography.

The rationale for treatment can therefore be understood. By giving venodilators the pulmonary venous pressure is reduced; diuretics enable the excess fluid to be excreted via the kidneys; ACE inhibitors inhibit angiotensin-II-mediated vasoconstriction and therefore reduce the workload of the heart; positive inotropes, such as dopamine and dobutamine, increase the contractility of the heart.

2.51 Schizophrenia   Answers: A B C D E

This question has been reported many times with virtually identical stems each time.

Many drugs of abuse produce a schizophreniform picture. These include amphetamines, opiates, and LSD. There is some suggestion that cannabis may also produce these symptoms.

Temporal lobe epilepsy is a great mimicker; it may produce auditory, olfactory or visual hallucinations.

In pregnancy there is an increased incidence of psychosis, both depressive and schizophrenic.

Hypoglycaemia may produce abnormal bizarre behaviour and is therefore marked 'true'. In this type of question the term 'schizophrenia' can be interpreted loosely as there is no reference to acute or chronic and therefore a broad range of symptoms is covered.

Acute schizophrenia may produce delusions, auditory hallucinations, thought disorders, abnormal affective responses and disordered behaviour. Schneider's first-rank symptoms for diagnosis include:

- thought insertion
- thought broadcasting
- hearing one's thoughts spoken out loud
- auditory hallucinations in the form of a running commentary
- auditory hallucinations in the form of voices discussing the patient in the third person
- feelings of passivity
- primary delusions.

Chronic schizophrenia causes slowness, apathy and social withdrawal as well as positive symptoms.

2.52 Hirsutism   Answers: A B C D E

This is a difficult question. We have used the harder stems from previous papers and put them into one question!

Hirsutism is an increase in body hair. Note that virilism is an increase in body hair in a male distribution. Virilism implies there is hirsutism but the other way round does not apply; a patient may be hirsute but not virilised, whereas a virilised patient is hirsute.

Signs of virilisation include a receding hair line, increased oiliness of the skin, breast atrophy, increased muscle bulk, clitoromegaly, increase in pubic hair and hair on the upper thighs, the lower abdomen, chest, breasts, and the moustache and beard areas. Fine hair on the face, arms and lower legs is not androgen dependent. Virilism is produced by excess androgens which may be adrenal in origin, for example congenital adrenal hyperplasia, or benign or malignant adrenal tumour. It may be ovarian in origin (for example, tumour, severe polycystic ovarian syndrome) or related to drug administration of androgens.

Hirsutism is caused by:

- all the above
- constitutional (endocrinology is normal, and it may be familial or racial)
- endocrine disorders (eg Cushing's syndrome, acromegaly, hyperthyroidism)
- metabolic conditions (eg porphyria cutanea tarda)
- drugs (eg minoxidil, phenytoin, diazoxide and corticosteroids)
- anorexia nervosa.

2.53 Abnormal speech   Answers: A B C D E

The production of speech is complex and involves pathways from the dominant motor cortex, pathways from the cerebellum for co-ordination of speech, temporal lobe for memory and the actual muscles involved in speech production, for example larynx, pharynx, tongue and facial muscles. The nerve supply to these muscles may be affected, as may the neuromuscular junction. Examples include lesions of the following:

- cerebral cortex (stroke)
- cerebellar (tumour, abscess, infarct, haemorrhage)
- central pathways (eg space-occupying lesions, demyelination)
- muscles (eg motor neurone disease)
- neuromuscular junction (eg myasthenia gravis)
- nerve supply (eg demyelination).

2.54 Ulcerative colitis   Answers: B C D E

Both ulcerative colitis and Crohn's disease have extra-gastrointestinal manifestations.

- Skin – erythema nodosum, pyoderma gangrenosum, vasculitis; note that dermatitis herpetiformis is associated with coeliac disease.
- Eyes – uveitis, episcleritis and conjunctivitis.
- Joints – monoarticular arthritis and sacroiliitis occur quite frequently in Crohn's disease. Ankylosing spondylitis occurs less commonly, whereas in ulcerative colitis ankylosing spondylitis is more common.
- Abdomen – fatty change of the liver is common in both Crohn's and ulcerative colitis and cirrhosis may occur in both; sclerosing cholangitis is more common in ulcerative colitis.
- Kidney and gall bladder stones occur very frequently in Crohn's disease but not ulcerative colitis.

All the above, apart from liver changes and renal and gall bladder stones are related to disease activity. In general, the presence of colitis in Crohn's disease causes more extra-gastrointestinal complications than if small-bowel lesions alone are present.

2.55 Heart sounds   Answers: A B C

The second heart sound is caused by closure of the aortic and pulmonary valves.

The left ventricle finishes emptying before the right heart and therefore the aortic component precedes the pulmonary component. Inspiration increases the venous return to the right heart further delaying right heart emptying and therefore closure of the pulmonary valve. This delay is physiological and is most commonly heard in children or young adults. It becomes abnormal (ie widely split in inspiration) when there is a further delay to right heart emptying, for example RBBB, pulmonary stenosis.

Left ventricular failure, aortic stenosis and LBBB delay emptying of the left heart and hence closure of the aortic valve. On inspiration the two sounds are close together but during expiration the right heart empties more quickly and the pulmonary valve closes earlier than the aortic valve, giving rise to reverse splitting.

The second heart sound is best heard with the diaphragm placed over the aortic or pulmonary area and the pulmonary component of the second heart sound is really only heard in the pulmonary area. Splitting in the mitral area is not physiological.

Fixed splitting only occurs in an ASD and is therefore pathognomonic. The aortic second sound is louder in systemic hypertension and when a hyperdynamic circulation is present. It is quiet in aortic stenosis because the valve is relatively immobile and in cardiac failure low blood flow also causes a quiet aortic component. Similarly, in pulmonary hypertension the pulmonary component of the second heart sound is loud and it is soft in pulmonary stenosis.

2.56 Tick-borne infection   Answer: D

Questions about infectious diseases are always extremely difficult and the amount of information to learn seems endless! It is worth knowing about malaria in some detail.

Insect transmission often appears in questions.

- Mosquitoes transmit malaria, dengue, yellow fever, filariasis
- Ticks/fleas carry typhus, Lyme disease, plague
- Flies transmit leishmaniasis, African trypanosomiasis, loiasis, onchocerciasis
- Bugs carry Chagas disease.

2.57 Statistics   Answers: C D E

The mode is the most frequently occurring value in a population. The median is the middle value when the values are ranked in order. The mean is sum of all the observed values divided by the number of values. In a normal distribution:

$$mean = mode = median$$

The standard deviation (SD) is a measure of the spread of a normally distributed population so that ±1 SD includes 68% of the population, ±2 SD includes 95% and ±3 SD includes 99% of the population.

2.58 Statistics   Answers: B C D

The standard error of the mean allows calculation of how accurate a sample mean is in estimating the mean of a population.

$$SE = SD/(n^{0.5})$$

where *n* is the number of values in the sample (not the square). From this a level of confidence can be calculated. The confidence is how close the sample mean is to the population mean. The sample mean ±2 SD is the confidence limit of the mean, ie 95% confident that the population mean lies within that range.

A *p* value of < 0.05 is usually taken to be representative of statistical significance.

The chi-squared test is used to test the difference between two independently derived proportions. It should be performed only on actual numbers of recurrences and not on percentages, proportions or means.

Student's *t*-test is useful for small samples with a normal distribution. Nonparametric tests are used to analyse data that do not conform to a normal distribution.

A type 1 error suggests that there is statistical significance when there is not and a type 2 error suggests a lack of significance when, in fact, there is significance.

2.59 Photosensitivity   Answers: A B D

The term 'photosensitivity' implies an abnormal sensitivity of the skin to light (both visible and UV). Implicit in this is an increased risk of skin cancer. The three important conditions producing photosensitivity are:

- SLE
- porphyria (all types except acute intermittent)
- pellagra.

By inducing the above conditions, drugs can also produce photosensitivity. For example, lupus may be induced by isoniazid, chlorpromazine, procainamide, hydralazine.

Pellagra may be induced by isoniazid. Oral contraceptives can produce lupus and porphyria. All the above induce photosensitivity indirectly.

Many drugs induce photosensitivity directly; for example, amiodarone, chlorpropamide, sulphonamides, quinine, psoralens. The drug is distributed systemically but interaction with sunlight is necessary so the rash only appears in sun-exposed areas.

2.60 Chorea   **Answers: A B C D**

Choreiform movements are sudden involuntary jerky movements. They are
due to a lesion of the corpus striatum. The abnormal movements occur more
distally compared to hemiballismus which tends to be unilateral and
involves the proximal joints and is caused by subthalamic lesions. Athetosis
produces a slow writhing movement distally and is due to a lesion of the
putamen.

The causes of chorea include:

- hereditary – benign hereditary chorea, Huntington's disease
- acquired endocrine – thyrotoxicosis, pregnancy
- connective tissue – SLE
- metabolic – Wilson's disease
- vascular – vasculitis, stroke
- infectious
  - bacterial: post-streptococcal infection may produce Sydenham's
    bacterial chorea, a major criterion for diagnosis of rheumatic fever
  - viral: viral encephalitis
- drugs – oral contraceptive pill, L-dopa, alcohol
- neoplasia – primary or secondary neoplasia.

BEST OF FIVE AND MULTIPLE CHOICE QUESTIONS PAPER 3

60 questions: time allowed 2½ hours

Best of Five Questions
Mark your answers with a tick (True) in the box provided.

3.1 A 39-year-old man with end-stage liver disease is admitted with a painful distended abdomen. Examination findings: generalised abdominal tenderness and ascites. Temperature 37.5°C. What treatment should be undertaken first?

❑ A Therapeutic paracentesis
❑ B Commence benzylpenicillin
❑ C Administer paracetamol
❑ D Commence cefotaxime
❑ E Commence spironolactone

3.2 A 36-year-old man is seen at outpatients clinic with the complaint of altered bowel habit. He reveals a 3-month history of increased frequency of motions of up to 8 times a day with PR blood on occasion. On examination: tender left iliac fossa. He was unable to tolerate a PR examination. Liver function tests forwarded by his GP revealed a raised alkaline phosphatase (ALP). Which one of the following findings on the autoantibody screen is most likely?

❑ A Raised anti-mitochondrial antibody (AMA)
❑ B Raised anti-smooth muscle antibody (ASMA)
❑ C Raised anti-endomysial
❑ D Negative
❑ E Raised anti-Jo

3.3 A 72-year-old lady with chronic congestive cardiac failure and renal impairment complains of a red, hot, swollen toe of sudden onset. This has occurred on a number of occasions. Her current medications include aspirin and azathioprine. The diagnosis is felt to be gout and she is prescribed colchicine. What is the most likely complaint from the patient?

☐ A A rash
☐ B Increased joint discomfort
☐ C Palpitations
☐ D Diarrhoea
☐ E Polydipsia

3.4 A 61-year-old man is admitted at the request of his concerned family due to increased confusion. This has occurred over the past 3 months and has become steadily worse. He was living independently and had been an active local Councillor. Now he is unable to identify his family members. Examination findings: pleasantly confused, intermittent jerky movements of both upper arms. The following investigations were performed. CT brain – normal. Dementia screen – normal. Which one of the following diagnostic tests will assist most in diagnosis?

☐ A Doppler ultrasound of carotids
☐ B Electroencephalogram
☐ C MRI brain
☐ D Muscle biopsy
☐ E Bone marrow biopsy

3.5 A 17-year-old patient with learning difficulties and poorly controlled epilepsy is admitted following a tonic–clonic seizure which resolved after the administration of lorazepam by a casualty officer. Twenty minutes later a further seizure occurred that again ceased with lorazepam. A further 10 min later another seizure takes place. What commonly would be the next step in the management of this patient?

☐ A Rectal diazepam
☐ B Admission to ICU
☐ C Paraldehyde
☐ D Topiramate
☐ E Fosphenytoin

3.6 A 32-year-old former air hostess attends general medical outpatient clinic with a host of constitutional symptoms. She has been extensively investigated previously but no diagnosis was found. She continues to insist she is unwell. She puts the following information she found on the internet in front of you and insists that you read it. Which one of the following is the only true disease–autoantibody association?

❏ A Myasthenia gravis: voltage-gated calcium channels
❏ B Polymyositis: anti-La
❏ C Wegener's granulomatosis: dsDNA
❏ D SLE: ANTI-Scl70
❏ E Chronic active hepatitis: anti-smooth muscle

3.7 A 28-year-old cyclist involved in a collision with a car requires placement of a central venous line (CVL). Which one of the following statements is most correct?

❏ A CVL placement is required for the administration of adrenaline
❏ B A femoral CVL is the site of choice
❏ C A CVL can be used for enteral feeding
❏ D A CVL should be routinely replaced fortnightly
❏ E A check radiograph is required on removal of a CVL

3.8 A 28-year-old man with valvular heart disease is admitted urgently with fever, increasing shortness of breath and a letter from his GP confirming the presence of a new murmur. On examination: harsh pan-systolic murmur + early diastolic murmur, Temperature 38.3°C. Bilateral, basal, fine crepitations. Which one of the following should take immediate priority?

❏ A Electrocardiogram
❏ B Echocardiogram
❏ C Administration of IV antibiotics
❏ D Throat swab
❏ E Administration of paracetamol

3.9 A 39-year-old lady attends her GP complaining of the development of painful, red areas on her shins. She has never been admitted to hospital and has not been abroad recently. She visited another GP in the practice recently and was commenced on a new tablet. Which medication listed is the likely culprit for this specific rash?

- ❏ A Atenolol
- ❏ B Fluoxetine
- ❏ C Microgynon 30
- ❏ D Fexofenadine
- ❏ E Minocycline

3.10 A 32-year-old former IV drug abuser is sent by his GP to outpatient clinic with deranged liver function tests (LFTs). He is asymptomatic, but on examination has a 4-cm hepar is noted. Blood tests reveal he is hepatitis C positive. The hepatitis C RNA viral load is significantly elevated. What investigation would be most important to guide future management?

- ❏ A HIV test
- ❏ B Ultrasound scan abdomen
- ❏ C Liver biopsy
- ❏ D CXR
- ❏ E Urine drug screening

3.11 A 50-year-old lady receives an invitation to attend for breast screening at her local hospital. Which one of the following statements with regard to breast screening is most accurate?

- ❏ A Screening is offered to 50- to 75-year-olds
- ❏ B Triple assessment is performed
- ❏ C Recall is on a yearly basis
- ❏ D Two mammogram views are routinely taken
- ❏ E Can only be performed on post-menopausal women

3.12   **A 59-year-old diabetic patient is admitted with dehydration. Over the next 48 h he deteriorates, having a seizure during the early hours of the morning. His serum biochemistry demonstrates a rising urea and creatinine. On day 3 his urea is 61 mmol/l and creatinine 899 μmol/l. His K⁺ is 6.0 mmol/l. CXR: heart size normal. Small bilateral pleural effusions. BP 168/98 mmHg. He is commenced on haemodialysis. What is the indication in this case for starting urgent dialysis?**

❑   A   An elevated serum potassium
❑   B   Severely elevated serum creatinine
❑   C   The occurrence of a seizure
❑   D   CXR findings
❑   E   Hypertension

3.13   **A 23-year old married shop assistant presents to casualty with a presumed seizure. This is the 2nd such event in the past 4 months and she was due to see a neurologist in a fortnight's time. CT brain was normal. EEG was normal, albeit not performed during the 'seizure' activity. Her doctor believes she has epilepsy and is keen to commence anticonvulsive therapy. She is sexually active and uses only condoms for protection. Which one of the following drugs would be most suitable for this particular patient?**

❑   A   Carbamazepine
❑   B   Sodium valproate
❑   C   Lamotrigine
❑   D   Phenytoin
❑   E   Levetiracetam

3.14 A 48-year-old lady attends her GP with lethargy, concerned as to whether she has reached the menopause. A screen of blood tests was performed with the positive findings being a Hb of 10.1 g/dl, MCV 108.2 fl and a B_{12} of 46 ng/l. Her only other complaint is occasional altered bowel habit. Which one of the following investigations would best help distinguish pernicious anaemia from malabsorption as the cause of her low B_{12}?

- ❏   A   PABA test
- ❏   B   Folic acid level
- ❏   C   Schilling's test
- ❏   D   Serum gastrin level
- ❏   E   C14 breath test

3.15 The ward nurses contact you because they are worried about a 46-year-old man admitted yesterday with jaundice. They found him in the linen cupboard apparently very disoriented. He explained he was looking for his luggage because he knew he needed to check out before midday. When you arrive he is wandering about very unsteadily, apparently still confused. On examination you find he has a tachycardia of 120 bpm and nystagmus. Which one of the following drugs would you give him first?

- ❏   A   Chlordiazepoxide
- ❏   B   Thiamine IM
- ❏   C   Haloperidol
- ❏   D   Propranolol
- ❏   E   Multivitamins

Multiple Choice Questions

Mark your answers with a tick (True) or a cross (False) in the box provided. Leave the box blank for 'Don't know'. Do not look at the answers until you have completed the whole question paper.

3.16 Features of Zollinger–Ellison syndrome include

- ❑ A Metabolic acidosis
- ❑ B Multiple peptic ulcers
- ❑ C High gastric acid levels
- ❑ D Low serum gastrin
- ❑ E Malignant potential

3.17 Neuropathic joints may occur in

- ❑ A Tuberculosis
- ❑ B Yaws
- ❑ C Leprosy
- ❑ D Syringomyelia
- ❑ E Tabes dorsalis

3.18 Recurrent renal stones may be due to

- ❑ A Hypoparathyroidism
- ❑ B High protein intake
- ❑ C Cystinuria
- ❑ D Crohn's disease
- ❑ E Hot climate

3.19 Positive test for rheumatoid factor occurs in

- ❑ A Reiter's syndrome
- ❑ B Chronic gout
- ❑ C Still's disease
- ❑ D Sjögren's syndrome
- ❑ E SLE

3.20   Recognised causes of pyrexia include

- ❏ A   Neuroleptic drugs
- ❏ B   Hodgkin's lymphoma
- ❏ C   Basal cell carcinoma
- ❏ D   Connective tissue disorders
- ❏ E   Hypothyroidism

3.21   The following commonly occur in heart failure

- ❏ A   A boot-shaped heart on chest radiograph
- ❏ B   Fine basal crepitations in the lung
- ❏ C   Pleural effusion
- ❏ D   Large pulmonary vessels
- ❏ E   Haemoptysis

3.22   The following imply that a bronchial carcinoma has metastasised

- ❏ A   Hyponatraemia
- ❏ B   Peripheral neuropathy
- ❏ C   Ptosis
- ❏ D   Ataxia
- ❏ E   Small-muscle wasting

3.23   Lower respiratory tract infections are more common in

- ❏ A   Crohn's disease
- ❏ B   Down's syndrome
- ❏ C   Emphysema
- ❏ D   Motor neurone disease
- ❏ E   Duchenne muscular dystrophy

3.24   Thrombocytopenia occurs in

- ❏ A   Chronic lymphocytic leukaemia
- ❏ B   Myelofibrosis
- ❏ C   SLE
- ❏ D   Prolonged aspirin therapy
- ❏ E   Acromegaly

3.25   Erectile dysfunction may result from

- ❏   A   A transurethral resection of the prostate
- ❏   B   Cimetidine therapy
- ❏   C   Depression
- ❏   D   Diabetes mellitus
- ❏   E   Chronic alcohol consumption

3.26   Chronic bronchitis may cause

- ❏   A   A raised arterial PCO_2
- ❏   B   A decreased arterial PO_2
- ❏   C   A raised haematocrit
- ❏   D   A raised hemidiaphragm on chest X-ray
- ❏   E   A raised pulmonary arterial pressure

3.27   The following cause a loud first heart sound

- ❏   A   Mitral stenosis
- ❏   B   Emphysema
- ❏   C   Anaemia
- ❏   D   Thin patient
- ❏   E   Heart failure

3.28   The following are causes of atrial fibrillation

- ❏   A   Chest infection
- ❏   B   Alcoholism
- ❏   C   Myocardial infarction
- ❏   D   Mitral valve regurgitation
- ❏   E   Myxoedema

3.29   The following may provide a clue to the aetiology of hypertension in a patient

- ❏   A   Systolic murmur near the midline of the back
- ❏   B   Episodic muscular weakness
- ❏   C   AV nipping in the retinal vessels
- ❏   D   Neurofibromas
- ❏   E   Tall R waves in V6

3.30   Jaundice producing dark urine occurs in

❏   A   Gilbert's syndrome
❏   B   Thalassaemia
❏   C   Carcinoma of the head of the pancreas
❏   D   Nitrazepam-induced jaundice
❏   E   Breast milk jaundice

3.31   In a cardiac arrest

❏   A   28% oxygen should be administered via a face mask until an
          anaesthetist arrives
❏   B   The ratio of cardiac compressions to ventilations is 30:2
❏   C   Adrenaline (1 mg) should be administered intravenously every 3–5
          min irrespective of the cardiac rhythm
❏   D   If the underlying rhythm is VF, 3 min of CPR should be performed
          between sequences of 3 shocks
❏   E   Atropine should be given in asystole

**3.32   Referral to an ophthalmologist is essential for all diabetic patients
         with**

❏   A   One microaneurysm
❏   B   One cotton wool spot
❏   C   One blot haemorrhage
❏   D   One hard exudate
❏   E   Maculopathy

3.33   Regarding ventricular fibrillation

❏   A   DC shock must not be attempted more than six times because of
          damage to the myocardium
❏   B   A central pulse may be present
❏   C   It may occur as a result of myocardial infarction
❏   D   The prognosis is better than for asystole
❏   E   Treatment should be abandoned after 5 min of ventricular
          fibrillation, as defibrillation after this time is unlikely to be
          successful

3.34   The following predispose to UTI

❏   A   Renal calculi
❏   B   Catheterisation
❏   C   Post-general anaesthetic
❏   D   Double ureter
❏   E   Being female

3.35   Causes of a round face include

❏   A   Cushing's syndrome
❏   B   Acromegaly
❏   C   Obesity
❏   D   Muscular dystrophy
❏   E   Nephrotic syndrome

3.36   In nephrotic syndrome

❏   A   There is an increased risk of infection
❏   B   Hypogammaglobulinaemia is diagnostic
❏   C   Venous thrombosis is common
❏   D   Children have a better outcome
❏   E   Renal failure will eventually occur

3.37   After pituitary ablation in a male the following must always be replaced

❏   A   Hydrocortisone
❏   B   Glucagon
❏   C   Thyroxine
❏   D   Testosterone
❏   E   Growth hormone

3.38   Patients with hypertension have an increased risk of

❏   A   Haemorrhagic stroke
❏   B   Embolic stroke
❏   C   Myocardial infarction
❏   D   Left ventricular failure
❏   E   Aortic stenosis

3.39   The following occur in nutritional rickets

❑   A   Raised serum alkaline phosphatase
❑   B   Lowered plasma calcium
❑   C   Raised serum phosphate
❑   D   Raised serum PTH
❑   E   Enlargement of the costochondral junction

3.40   Swelling of the arm may be caused by

❑   A   SVC obstruction
❑   B   Breast surgery
❑   C   Radiotherapy
❑   D   Ipsilateral stroke
❑   E   Aortic dissection

3.41   Asbestos exposure may cause

❑   A   Left ventricular failure
❑   B   Bronchial carcinoma
❑   C   Lung fibrosis
❑   D   Mesothelioma
❑   E   Pleural and peritoneal plaques

3.42   Bone metastases are commonly produced by the following cancers

❑   A   Prostate
❑   B   Thyroid
❑   C   Breast
❑   D   Ovary
❑   E   Brain

3.43   Weight loss of over 6.5 kg in 2 months may be due to

❑   A   Depression
❑   B   Anxiety
❑   C   Bronchial adenoma
❑   D   Hyperthyroidism
❑   E   Diabetes mellitus

3.44   Causes of clinically significant weight gain include

❏   A   Nephrotic syndrome
❏   B   Bronchial carcinoma
❏   C   Pelvic malignancy
❏   D   Congestive cardiac failure
❏   E   Diabetes insipidus

3.45   Causes of absent ankle jerk reflexes include

❏   A   Old age
❏   B   Diabetes mellitus
❏   C   Syphilis
❏   D   Motor neurone disease
❏   E   Parkinson's disease

3.46   A bowed tibia may be due to

❏   A   Paget's disease
❏   B   Osteoporosis
❏   C   Rickets
❏   D   Syphilis
❏   E   Rheumatoid arthritis

3.47   Polyuria and polydipsia may be due to

❏   A   Hypokalaemia
❏   B   Hypocalcaemia
❏   C   Diabetes mellitus
❏   D   Acute renal failure
❏   E   Diabetes insipidus

3.48   A generalised change in skin colour occurs with

❏   A   Pernicious anaemia
❏   B   Haemochromatosis
❏   C   Hypercarotinaemia
❏   D   Carbon monoxide poisoning
❏   E   Lead poisoning

3.49   Vomiting may result from

❏ A   Hip surgery
❏ B   Low serum potassium
❏ C   Opiate use
❏ D   Caecal carcinoma
❏ E   Ménière's disease

3.50   Features suggestive of a diagnosis of irritable bowel syndrome include

❏ A   Weight loss
❏ B   Change in bowel habit
❏ C   Small amounts of blood from the rectum
❏ D   Improvement on a gluten-free diet
❏ E   Dysphagia

3.51   The following diseases are paired with appropriate investigations

❏ A   Sarcoid – thallium scan
❏ B   Myocardial ischaemia – gallium scan
❏ C   Left ventricular function – MUGA scan
❏ D   Lung metastases – MRI
❏ E   Caecal carcinoma – ultrasound

3.52   Scalp hair may decrease with

❏ A   Hypothyroidism
❏ B   Hypopituitarism
❏ C   Minoxidil tablets
❏ D   Stress
❏ E   Cisplatin

3.53   Which of the following are good screening tests

❏ A   Faecal occult bloods for a GI malignancy
❏ B   Genetic tests for breast cancer
❏ C   Random cortisol for Cushing's syndrome
❏ D   Resting ECG for asymptomatic coronary artery disease
❏ E   CA125 for ovarian carcinoma

3.54   **The following statements are true concerning the prevalence of a disease**

❏   A   It is determined from a longitudinal study
❏   B   It is determined from cross-sectional studies
❏   C   It depends on the duration of the illness
❏   D   It is equal to the mortality rate when the case fatality ratio is high
❏   E   For asthma it is 25%

3.55   **A low serum iron and low total iron binding capacity may occur with**

❏   A   Rheumatoid arthritis
❏   B   Anaemia of chronic disease
❏   C   Hereditary spherocytosis
❏   D   Iron deficiency
❏   E   Pernicious anaemia

3.56   **A raised faecal fat may occur with**

❏   A   Ulcerative colitis
❏   B   Subtotal villous atrophy
❏   C   Gallstones
❏   D   Chronic pancreatitis
❏   E   Gastrin-secreting tumour

3.57   **Pleural effusion occurs with**

❏   A   Oesophagitis
❏   B   Tuberculosis
❏   C   Rheumatoid arthritis
❏   D   Aortic valve replacement
❏   E   Rheumatic fever

3.58   **Generalised lymphadenopathy may be caused by**

❏   A   Glandular fever
❏   B   Mumps
❏   C   Syphilis
❏   D   Multiple myeloma
❏   E   HIV infection

3.59   The following are examined in order to certify death

- ❏   A   Jugular venous pressure
- ❏   B   Heart sounds
- ❏   C   Radial pulse
- ❏   D   Response to external stimuli
- ❏   E   Breath sounds

3.60   Angina pectoris may be precipitated by

- ❏   A   Anaemia
- ❏   B   A large meal
- ❏   C   Watching a violent television programme
- ❏   D   Thyroxine, acute
- ❏   E   Myocardial infarction

———————————— **END** ————————————

**Go over your answers until your time is up. Correct answers
and teaching notes are overleaf**

BEST OF FIVE AND MULTIPLE CHOICE QUESTIONS PAPER 3
Answers

The correct answer options for each question are given below.

3.1	D	3.31	B C E
3.2	D	3.32	B E
3.3	D	3.33	C D
3.4	B	3.34	A B C D E
3.5	E	3.35	A C E
3.6	E	3.36	A C D
3.7	A	3.37	A C D
3.8	C	3.38	A B C D
3.9	C	3.39	A B D
3.10	C	3.40	A B C D
3.11	D	3.41	B C D E
3.12	C	3.42	A B C
3.13	C	3.43	A D E
3.14	C	3.44	A C D
3.15	B	3.45	A B C D
3.16	A B C E	3.46	A C D
3.17	B C D E	3.47	A C E
3.18	B C D E	3.48	A C D
3.19	D E	3.49	A C D E
3.20	A B D	3.50	All false
3.21	B C D E	3.51	C
3.22	All false	3.52	A B D E
3.23	B C D E	3.53	E
3.24	A B C	3.54	B C
3.25	A C D E	3.55	A B
3.26	A B C E	3.56	B D E
3.27	A C D	3.57	B C D
3.28	A B C D	3.58	A C E
3.29	A B D	3.59	B D E
3.30	C D	3.60	A B C D

BEST OF FIVE AND MULTIPLE CHOICE QUESTIONS PAPER 3
Answers

3.1 D: Commence cefotaxime

Spontaneous bacterial peritonitis (SBP) may occur in any patient with ascites. Those with end-stage liver disease with poor synthetic function develop ascites easily and are susceptible to spontaneous infection. These patients are also relatively immunocompromised as a consequence of their underlying disease. This condition may present itself both subjectively and objectively with generalised abdominal discomfort. This group of patients have the potential to become unwell quickly and there is a high mortality rate. Immediate treatment is warranted. This often means 'covering' the patient with antibiotics first – the drug of choice being cefotaxime. Ideally a *diagnostic paracentesis* is performed promptly and cefotaxime given immediately afterwards. Once SPB has been excluded or treated consideration may be given to the merits of therapeutic paracentesis.

3.2 D: Negative

A clear understanding of the wide range of autoantibodies and their associations is important. This is a common and recurring theme in medical exams. The results should always be interpreted in the context of the clinical features, as the sensitivity and specificity are variable. This question also demonstrates another popular form of questioning in establishing the candidates' understanding of disease association and ability to think laterally. This patient's description is hinting at inflammatory bowel disease (ulcerative colitis) and its association with primary sclerosing cholangitis (PSC). In this condition immunologically mediated inflammation of the bile ducts causes stricturing within the biliary tree best demonstrated on ERCP and magnetic resonance cholangiopancreatography (MRCP). There is no strong link with a specific autoantibody. An isolated ALP rise is often observed. This should not be confused with primary biliary cirrhosis (PBC) in which the antimitochondrial antibody is typically raised. Some of the typical antibody associations are shown below.

Antibody	Disease association
Antimitochondrial antibody	Primary biliary cirrhosis
Anti-smooth muscle antibody	Chronic active hepatitis
Anti-endomysial, gliadin, transglutamase	Coeliac disease
Anti-gastric parietal cell and anti-intrinsic factor	Pernicious anaemia
Anti-dsDNA	SLE
pANCA	Churg–Strauss
cANCA	Wegener's granulomatosis
Anti-centromere	Limited scleroderma

3.3 D: Diarrhoea

It is routine to manage patients with multiple medical co-morbidities on a concoction of medications. In many instances the poly-pharmacy itself may be contributing to a patient's symptoms or adding to significant challenges in treating one condition without detriment to the other.

The standard treatment for acute gout is non-steroidal anti-inflammatory drugs (NSAIDs). With renal impairment and congestive cardiac failure (CCF) the use of NSAIDs for acute gout is contraindicated. It may worsen renal impairment. It has a propensity to causes fluid retention and so worsen CCF. Colchicine has been used as an alternative – it is however notorious for causing gastrointestinal side-effects including diarrhoea. Prophylactic therapy for this patient is likewise difficult. There is a major interaction between azathioprine and the potential prophylactic treatment for gout – allopurinol. Allopurinol is a xanthine-oxidase inhibitor. It prevents the breakdown of purines which produces uric acid. Azathioprine is metabolised into mercaptopurine and therefore its breakdown is slowed down when co-prescribed with allopurinol. It should therefore be replaced with an alternative agent or the dose of azathioprine reduced to take into account the effects of allopurinol on its metabolism.

3.4 B: Electroencephalogram

The essential history to extract from this question is one of rapid cognitive decline with associated myoclonic jerks in a patient in their sixties. Furthermore, the majority of investigations into a confusional state have been undertaken and revealed no positive findings. This clinical scenario is suggestive of sporadic Creutzfeldt–Jakob disease (sCJD) – a neuro-degenerative condition. The key investigations to support this clinical diagnosis are lumbar puncture and an electroencephalogram (EEG). Definitive diagnosis can only be made from biopsy, which is invariably undertaken at post-mortem. Lumbar puncture will allow cerebrospinal fluid (CSF) to be analysed for protein 14-3-3. This is time consuming and is not included in the stems listed. Furthermore, 14-3-3 is a normal neuronal protein and may be released into the CSF in response to a variety of neuronal insults. EEG is the test of choice. If positive this will classically demonstrate generalised bi- or triphasic periodic sharp wave complexes appearing with a frequency of around 1–2 per second.

3.5 E: Fosphenytoin

Epilepsy is largely a manageable condition. The majority of epileptics are well controlled on oral anticonvulsants with only the occasional seizure. The vast majority of seizures will self resolve. These patients are unlikely to reach hospital attention. Of those patients in whom a single fit does not self resolve within several minutes a common approach, if available, is to use benzodiazepines. This may be rectal diazepam or intravenous lorazepam. It can be given in increments until the seizure resolves. If a further seizure occurs soon after it may again be appropriate to use further benzodi- azepines providing consideration is given to the possibility of causing respi- ratory depression.

However, if another seizure takes place other drugs should be given – IV fosphenytoin being the most recognized. Fifty percent of patients who do not resolve seizure activity to initial benzodiazepine treatment will respond with the addition of fosphenytoin. At this point it would be appropriate to inform ICU of a potential patient with status epilepticus. Paraldehyde could be used instead of fosphenytoin but is far less popular in contemporary adult medicine. Fosphenytoin (a pro-drug of phenytoin) is preferable if available. It can be given more rapidly and fewer reactions have been noted. ECG monitoring is required. A loading dose is administered, followed by an intravenous infusion.

3.6 E: Chronic active hepatitis: anti-smooth muscle

With the growing use of the internet and a shift in control in doctor–patient relationships it is not at all uncommon to be presented with vast quantities of information from patients. The information may have been acquired from websites with no clinical evidence to support the data and demanding ques- tions are asked by patients and their relatives.

The true association is that of chronic active hepatitis (CAH) (a form of autoimmune hepatitis) and anti-smooth muscle antibody. A disease may have more than one autoantibody associated. CAH is also linked with an anti-liver-kidney-microsomal (LKM1) antibody. Likewise a disease with different clinical entities may have different autoantibodies. Diffuse sclero-derma is associated with anti-scleroderma 70 (anti-Scl70) whilst limited scleroderma is associated with anti-centromere antibody.

Myasthenia gravis	Acetylcholine receptor
Eaton–Lambert myasthenic syndrome	Voltage-gated calcium channels
Polymyositis	Anti-Jo
Wegener's granulomatosis	cANCA (anti-neutrophil cytoplasmic antibody)
SLE	dsDNA

The strength of association is variable and should always be interpreted in the context of the clinical history.

3.7 A: CVL placement is required for the administration of adrenaline

Central venous lines (CVL) are placed in three common locations: internal jugular, subclavian and femoral veins. The site of choice in terms of the lowest line sepsis rate is subclavian, although the complication risk is higher. Femoral lines are most susceptible to infection due to the flora within the groin area. Although the risk–benefit of a CVL increases with the age of the line a specified time limit is uncommon and certainly is not as lengthy as fortnightly. Consideration of the age of all lines should be made on daily review within the ICU/HDU environment. A check radiograph for placement is recommended on insertion of both subclavian and internal jugular lines – to confirm correct placement within the superior vena cava and to exclude a procedural pneumothorax.

Uses of central venous lines:

- Administration of drugs – including inotropes such as **adrenaline**
- Parenteral nutrition
- Blood products
- Fluids.

3.8 C: Administration of IV antibiotics

Subacute bacterial endocarditis (SBE) requires rapid diagnosis and treatment. An existing or prosthetic valve may be destroyed if left untreated. Those with pre-existing heart or valve abnormalities are more susceptible and patient education regarding prophylactic antibiotics before a number of 'routine' procedures is required, This includes dental treatment outside of hospital. One should always suspect and aim to exclude SBE in any patient with known valve disease and pyrexia. A new or changing murmur likewise should be viewed with huge suspicion. All of the stems in reality are important in the treatment of this patient and in an ideal world would be performed immediately and simultaneously. ECHO is clearly required for proven diagnosis – a transoesophageal (TOE) may be required if transthoracic ECHO is equivocal. Three sets of blood cultures over a 24-h period are required in order that the antibiotic regime is effective against the causative organism. However, it is essential that IV antibiotics are commenced at the earliest possible opportunity to limit valve destruction. An empirical regime of low dose gentamicin (1mg/kg) 8 hourly and benzylpenicillin 2.4 6 hourly may be used until microbiological advice suggests any alternative.

3.9 C: Microgynon 30

Erythema nodosum is a panniculitis. It typically occurs on the anterior aspect of the lower legs (shins) and is it raised in nature (nodular). Its characteristic feature is that it is *painful*, unlike most other rashes in this distribution. Drugs are a recognised cause of erythema nodusum, and include the oral contraceptive pill. Other medications recognised to cause this rash include penicillins and sulphonamides. Given the association with both tuberculosis and sarcoidosis it is commonplace to perform a chest radiograph at diagnosis in an attempt to exclude these serious causes of erythema nodosum.

Causes of erythema nodosum:

- Idiopathic (COMMONEST)
- Tuberculosis
- Inflammatory bowel disease
- Sarcoidosis
- Drugs, including the oral contraceptive pill (eg, Microgynon 30)
- Infection (eg streptococcal throat infection)
- Pregnancy.

3.10 C: Liver biopsy

Hepatitis C may be acute or more often a chronic disease caused by the hepatitis C RNA virus. It may be acquired from blood or sexual intercourse. This includes shared needles through intravenous drug use as well as from contaminated blood products. In the UK blood products are now routinely screened for hepatitis C. Patients are often asymptomatic in the initial stages of the disease. The virus is 'cleared' by the body's own immune system in a small percentage. For the majority it remains and continues to cause progressive damage to the liver. Liver failure requiring transplantation is a distinct possibility if left untreated. A regime of ribavarin and pegylated inter-feron-alpha is used for 6–12 months with the aim of eliminating hepatitis C RNA from the blood. However this treatment does not guarantee clearance (the success depends on the genotype of the virus) and has significant side-effects. The most important side-effects include leucopenia and anaemia, which may require discontinuation of the treatment or co-prescription of erythropoietin and the use of granulocyte stimulating factor (GSF).

In order to assess the merits of treatment the degree of liver damage needs to be assessed. For this liver biopsy is required. The necro-inflammatory and fibrosis scores guide the clinician. For those with established fibrosis the risk of developing hepatocellular carcinoma (HCC) should not be ignored. Enrolment in a 6-monthly ultrasound screening programme is recommended. Alpha-1-fetoprotein should also be monitored, given its association with this primary liver tumour.

3.11 D: Two mammogram views are routinely taken

The UK Breast Screening Service offers three-yearly screening of women aged between 50 and 70 years of age. It involves taking two views of the breast (cranio-caudal and lateral oblique) by mammography. Mammography is a specialised form of plain radiography used exclusively for breast imaging. Those under the age of 50 years are not invited as trying to observe small abnormalities in the breast is less reliable. This is because the more glandular nature of the young breast is very similar to the density of tumour whereas the fattier breast of an older, largely post-menopausal woman is of a different density. Triple assessment is the procedure under which any women found to have a breast lump, either by screening or otherwise, undergoes. It comprises of imaging (mammography ± ultra-sound), clinical assessment and histopathology (biopsy).

> **Tripe assessment = Clinical assessment + Imaging + Histopathology**

3.12 C: The occurrence of a seizure

There are a limited number of indications for urgent dialysis in the treatment of acute renal failure (ARF). In this case symptomatic severe uraemia is the indication. The patient has a very high urea of 61 mmol/l and has developed a seizure as a consequence.

Indications for urgent renal dialysis in acute renal failure:

- Hyperkalaemia (K^+ >6.5 mmol/l)
- Pulmonary oedema
- Profound acidosis (pH<7.1)
- Severe uraemia with symptoms, including pericarditis.

3.13 C: Lamotrigine

For an adult with generalised epilepsy carbamazepine and sodium valproate are first-line agents. In women of childbearing age (regardless of stated contraception) the choice of agents is different. Sodium valproate has an association with neural tube defects. One should be especially careful for those taking more than one antiepileptic as combination therapy has potentially worse outcomes. The UK Epilepsy and Pregnancy Registry (http: //www.epilepsyand-pregnancy.co.uk/) aids the clinician in this respect. Lamotrigine monotherapy has proved to be an excellent choice in childbearing women.

3.14 C: Schilling's Test

The Schilling's test is used to distinguish between different causes of vitamin B_{12} deficiency.

Normally vitamin B_{12} is absorbed in the terminal ileum, but only after being bound to intrinsic factor (a protein) secreted by the gastric parietal cells of the stomach. A problem in any part of this chain may result in vitamin B_{12} deficiency.

As part of the test patients are given two doses of vitamin B_{12}.

1. Intramuscular B_{12} (non radioactively labelled)
2. Radioactively labelled oral B_{12}.

Urine is then collected over a 24-h period to measure the amount of radioactive vitamin B_{12} which is excreted in the urine. Normally, 10% or more of the oral dose is found in the urine (the remainder is absorbed). In malabsorption a smaller proportion will be found in the urine. If the proportion is reduced in the urine then a second stage to the test is performed.

The test is repeated with oral radioactive vitamin B_{12} and oral intrinsic factor. If the proportion of vitamin B_{12} in the urine is then normal the lack of intrinsic factor is the cause. This is usually due to pernicious anaemia, whereby autoantibodies against either the gastric parietal cells or intrinsic factor itself cause a deficiency of intrinsic factor. Without this vitamin B_{12} cannot be properly absorbed.

If the proportion of radioactive vitamin B_{12} in the urine remains abnormal the problem lies in the terminal ileum, and causes include bacterial overgrowth.

3.15 B: Thiamine IM

This man has Wernicke's encephalopathy, a disorder caused by thiamine deficiency. In the UK it is usually seen in alcohol withdrawal. It is characterised by the triad of: ophthalmoplegia, confusion and ataxia. Left untreated, it can develop into Korsakoff's syndrome (amnesic disorder) with lasting and profound memory impairment. Parenteral thiamine replacement is required. Intramuscular thiamine (Pabrinex®) is usually preferred to intravenous thiamine as it carries a lower risk of anaphylaxis. This should be given in a setting where resuscitation facilities are available. Thiamine is also given prophylactically in alcohol withdrawal.

Benzodiazepines (eg chlordiazepoxide) are given in alcohol withdrawal to reduce the risk of seizures as well as subjective discomfort and are probably indicated here. However, the priority must be to treat the cause of encephalopathy. Benzodiazepines also adequately treat/prevent milder forms of perceptual disturbance often seen in the alcohol withdrawal syndrome, but antipsychotic medication such as haloperidol will be required for frank hallucinations. Oral vitamins are given to patients during and after detoxification to supplement thiamine and compensate for poor nutrition.

3.16 Zollinger–Ellison syndrome   Answers: A B C E

Zollinger–Ellison syndrome is due to a gastrin-secreting tumour that usually arises from G cells in the pancreas. The secretion of gastrin is autonomous and a raised serum gastrin occurs. This in turn produces high levels of acid with the following consequences:

- multiple duodenal ulceration
- metabolic acidosis
- diarrhoea (stimulated by the low pH in the upper intestine).

Patients may present with diarrhoea, or abdominal pain, ulceration and the complications of ulceration, such as haemorrhage and perforation. Omeprazole is the mainstay of treatment although surgery to remove the primary tumour may be performed. The tumour is malignant but slow growing. The syndrome may be part of the wider multiple endocrine neoplasia (MEN) syndrome involving pituitary tumours, parathyroid adenomas and pancreatic tumours.

3.17 Neuropathic joints   Answers: B C D E

A neuropathic or Charcot's joint is a grossly disorganised but painless joint. It is caused by loss of sensory nerve supply of a joint and hence loss of protective pain sensation. The joint is characteristically swollen with abnormal but painless movement. Causes include tabes dorsalis, syringomyelia, diabetes mellitus, subacute combined degeneration, leprosy and yaws. Tuberculosis may cause painful destruction of a joint.

3.18 Renal stones   Answers: B C D E

Important causes of urinary tract stone formation include dehydration; for example, living in a hot climate, multiple myeloma or prolonged illness. Metabolic disturbances include hypercalcaemia (eg hyperparathyroidism, sarcoidosis, malignancy); increased oxalate, such as in Crohn's disease; increased uric acid levels, for example a high protein diet may cause uric acid deposition in the joints causing gout or in the kidney causing stones; cystinuria – produces cystine stones.

Note that stones can cause infection and vice versa.

Stones may also be caused by renal disease, such as renal tubular acidosis.

3.19 Rheumatoid factor   Answers: D E

A positive test for rheumatoid factor may occur in rheumatoid arthritis, Sjögren's syndrome, SLE, systemic sclerosis, mixed connective tissue disease and polymyositis.

3.20 Pyrexia   Answers: A B D

There are many causes of pyrexia and, although it is tempting to think of infection as the cause, the wide differential must be remembered. Causes include:

- infection
- inflammation (eg inflammatory bowel disease)
- malignancy – lymphomas, leukaemias and carcinoma of the liver, pancreas and kidney particularly produce fever, but any disseminated malignancy may also do so. Localised skin tumour, such as basal cell carcinoma, is unlikely to cause a fever unless there is coexisting infection
- connective tissue disorders (eg SLE, rheumatoid arthritis)
- vasculitis (eg polyarteritis nodosa, sarcoidosis)
- drugs – neuroleptic drugs, such as chlorpromazine, may cause neuroleptic malignant syndrome which causes a very high fever; allergic drug reactions will also produce a fever
- aspirin overdose can produce a hyperpyrexia
- endocrine (eg thyroid storm – hypothyroidism produces hypothermia)
- hypothalamic lesions – the central control of temperature is here.

3.21 Heart failure   Answers: B C D E
(See also the answer to Paper 2, Question 2.50.)

As the left ventricle fails, blood is not pumped out of the heart effectively, causing an increase in pressure in the left ventricle. This is transmitted back to the left atrium and then the pulmonary veins.

On a chest X-ray this can be seen, at first, as an increase in heart size. An increase in both the size and number of upper lobe blood vessels then occurs and as the pressure increases further, fluid leaks into the lung interstitium where it appears as fluid in the horizontal fissure, septal lines, etc, or as a pleural effusion. Further pressure rises causes fluid in the alveoli, ie alveolar oedema.

The raised pulmonary venous pressure may cause more vessels to rupture producing haemoptysis (usually small). As the left ventricle fails it enlarges and on chest X-ray the cardiothoracic ratio increases. However, nothing further can be said about the shape of the heart; a boot-shaped heart occurs in Fallot's tetralogy.

3.22 Bronchial carcinoma   Answers: All false
This question illustrates the wide variety of effects that a bronchial malignancy may have.

Compression, effusion or obstruction:
- Nerve compression
  - Cervical sympathetic nerve – producing Horner's syndrome
  - Recurrent laryngeal nerve damage – producing voice hoarseness
  - Phrenic nerve damage – producing an elevated hemidiaphragm
  - T1 nerve damage – leading to small-muscle wasting
- Vessel compression
  - Artery or vein (eg superior vena caval obstruction)
- Pleural effusion
  - Empyema
- Airway obstruction
  - Stridor
  - Collapse
  - Distal infection
  - Air trapping

Metastases:
- Discrete lung metastases or hilar node metastases
  - Brain, liver, adrenal glands, bone

Non-metastatic effects:
- Hormone secretion – especially oat cell tumours
  - ACTH (Cushing's syndrome), PT (hypercalcaemia), ADH (hyponatraemia)
- Skin changes (eg erythema gyratum repens)
- Hypotrophic pulmonary osteoarthropathy and clubbing
- Neuropathy, myopathy, cachexia, weight loss
- Ataxia – this may be a paraneoplastic phenomenon and therefore does not imply cerebellar metastases, although these should also be considered.

3.23 Lower respiratory tract infections   Answers: B C D E

An increase in incidence of lower respiratory tract infections is seen in:
- Primary lung disease (eg bronchiectasis, bronchitis, emphysema).
- Cardiac disease (eg septal defects, pulmonary hypertension; Down's syndrome patients have a higher incidence of these defects).
- Neuromuscular disorders, eg motor neurone disease – these patients are at risk of aspiration due to bulbar damage and also have difficulty ventilating their lungs due to thoracic wall muscle involvement and diaphragmatic paresis. In myasthenia gravis, fatigue may prevent adequate coughing.
- Mechanical restriction to adequate lung ventilation; for example, Duchenne muscular dystrophy, polio, ankylosing spondylitis and conditions producing a kyphoscoliosis.

3.24 Thrombocytopenia   Answers: A B C

Thrombocytopenia is defined as a platelet count of less than $150 \times 10^9/l$. Causes include:
- Decreased production
  - Bone marrow failure due to drugs or malignancy, such as leukaemia
  - Megaloblastic anaemia (eg vitamin B_{12} or folate deficiency) results in decreased marrow function
  - Uraemia has a deleterious effect on marrow, producing thrombocytopenia
  - Alcohol appears to have numerous effects on bone marrow, including direct suppression of function by a toxic effect
  - B_{12}/folate deficiency leads to megaloblastic anaemia
  - Cirrhosis produces portal hypertension and splenomegaly, the latter causing thrombocytopenia
  - Viral infections (eg measles, CMV) can inhibit platelet production.

- Decreased survival
  - For example, immunological autoantibodies are formed against the platelets resulting in their premature destruction; this occurs in conditions such as SLE, chronic lymphatic leukaemia and ITP (idiopathic thrombocytopenic purpura). Some mechanisms of drug-mediated thrombocytopenia are thought to be autoimmune (eg heparin, sulphonamides, quinine).
- Increased consumption
  - DIC (disseminated intravascular coagulation); sequestration in the spleen (eg liver cirrhosis and portal hypertension); massive haemorrhage.

Note that aspirin causes platelet dysfunction but not thrombocytopenia; other drugs with effects on platelets similar to aspirin include indometacin and streptokinase.

Note that platelet dysfunction may occur despite a normal or even high platelet count. For example, in renal failure and hepatic failure the platelet count may be reduced as mentioned above, or it may be normal with a qualitative defect. In myeloproliferative disorders thrombocythemia may occur, ie an increase in platelets occurs, but the platelet function is abnormal.

3.25 Erectile dysfunction
Answers: A C D E

Erectile dysfunction (impotence) may result from damage to the nerve or vessels supplying the penis. Nerve damage may follow transurethral resection of the prostate (TURP) and patients must be warned of this. Drug therapy, for example with beta-blockers, alpha-blockers and thiazide diuretics, may also cause this.

In diabetes mellitus, autonomic nerve damage may occur; the parasympathetic nervous system is responsible for erection and sympathetic nerve for ejaculation. Chronic alcohol consumption will also cause erectile impotence. The higher centres also have an important role and anxiety or depression may produce impotence.

Cystic fibrosis causes infertility in males but not impotence.

3.26 Chronic bronchitis
Answers: A B C E

Patients with chronic bronchitis are often hypoxic. Mucus plugging in the airways and damage to their walls, together with loss of elastic recoil (as in emphysema), producing early closure of the airways during expiration, all contribute to this hypoxia. Unless the patient can hyperventilate, the PCO_2 will also rise, producing a respiratory acidosis. The kidneys retain bicarbonate to normalise the pH so in the chronic state a patient with chronic bronchitis and PCO_2 retention has a raised PCO_2, raised plasma bicarbonate and normal pH (ie a compensated respiratory acidosis).

Hypoxia has an important effect; it acts as a stimulus for erythropoietin production by the kidney and polycythaemia produces a rise in haematocrit. The latter can be such a problem as to warrant regular venesection in order to prevent complications such as stroke.

Hypoxia in an area of lung causes vasoconstriction of the blood vessels in that area. This is a protective response in that it diverts blood flow from areas of poor ventilation to those that are better ventilated. However, in the long term, chronic vasoconstriction produces changes in the vessel walls causing a rise in pulmonary arterial pressure. This can eventually lead to cor pulmonale (ie right heart failure secondary to lung disease).

A raised hemidiaphragm on a chest X-ray should not be attributed to chronic bronchitis alone. A coexisting lung lesion should be suspected.

3.27 Heart sounds   Answers: A C D
The first heart sound is loud in:

- thin patients
- hyperdynamic circulation (eg thyrotoxicosis or severe anaemia)
- mitral stenosis
- short PR interval.

The heart sound is soft in obese patients; in pericardial effusion or tamponade; in emphysema; in cardiac failure when the PR interval is long and in mitral valve regurgitation (valve closure produces the first heart sound and therefore if the valve does not close properly the heart sound is quiet).

3.28 Atrial fibrillation   Answers: A B C D

There are many causes of atrial fibrillation; the most important ones are ischaemic heart disease, rheumatic heart disease and thyrotoxicosis. The important causes can be considered under the following headings:

- Cardiac causes – valve disease (eg mitral valve disease – whatever the cause); conduction abnormality (eg Wolf–Parkinson–White syndrome); cardiomyopathy; pericardial disease, pericarditis.

- Lung disease – carcinoma of the bronchus; pulmonary embolus; pneumonia.
- Metabolic thyrotoxicosis; alcohol abuse – acute and chronic.
- Lone atrial fibrillation is the term used to describe atrial fibrillation when no cause is discovered; this accounts for about 5% of cases.

3.29 Hypertension
Answers: A B D

Hypertension may be essential (90%) or secondary (10%). This question refers to causes of secondary hypertension.

Renal causes include chronic glomerulonephritis and polycystic renal disease. Renal artery stenosis due to fibromuscular hyperplasia or atheroma may also cause hypertension. Renal causes are the most common cause of secondary hypertension.

Endocrine causes include Conn's syndrome, in which episodic muscular weakness occurs due to hypokalaemia. Other symptoms include tetany and nocturia. Phaeochromocytomas produce excess catecholamines that cause palpitations, tremor, sweating, headache, flushing, etc. Hypertension may be intermittent or constant and postural hypotension may be present (another common question). Tachycardia, bradycardia and other arrhythmias may occur. Flushing, fever and glycosuria are also features. Phaeochromocytoma may occur in association with other conditions, for example neurofibromatosis, Cushing's syndrome, acromegaly and hyper-parathyroidism are also causes of secondary hypertension.

Cardiac causes include coarctation of the aorta. A systolic murmur near the midline of the back occurs.

Note that the question refers to the causes of hypertension and not the consequences, which include retinal changes and ECG changes due to cardiac enlargement.

3.30 Jaundice
Answers: C D

Dark urine in jaundice implies that there is an obstruction to conjugated bilirubin entering the bowel. This results in overspill of conjugated bilirubin into the urine producing a dark colour. Causes of obstructive jaundice include gallstones, biliary tract tumours, sclerosing cholangitis and carcinoma of the head of the pancreas. These all cause extra-hepatic obstruction. Intra-hepatic biliary obstruction can occur with drugs such as nitrazepam.

When unconjugated bilirubin is in excess it is excreted into the urine. It has no colour, hence the term acholuric jaundice. Causes of this include:

- deficiency of conjugating enzymes, eg Gilbert's syndrome
- relative lack of functioning enzymes, eg infants who are breast-fed may develop physiological jaundice
- increase in red cell products, eg thalassaemia.

In the haemoglobinopathies the abnormal red cells are broken down more quickly, producing an increase in red cell products.

3.31 Cardiac arrest
Answers: B C E

The immediate management of the airway in a cardiorespiratory arrest is to call the resuscitation team, extend the neck, clear the oropharynx, insert a Guedel airway and start bag-valve mask or mouth-to-mask ventilation. 100% oxygen should be administered as soon as possible. The lungs should be ventilated twice after every 30th cardiac compression irrespective of the number of resuscitators.

When there is no cardiac output, whatever the underlying cardiac rhythm, 1 mg adrenaline should be given every 3–5 min.

CPR should be as continuous as possible. If the patient is in ventricular fibrillation that has not responded to one DC shock, 2 min of CPR should be undertaken before cardioversion is attempted again.

Atropine should be administered in asystole or bradycardic electromechanical dissociation (EMD).

3.32 Diabetic eye disease
Answers: B E

Referral to an ophthalmologist must be made for all diabetic patients with maculopathy, new vessels (an emergency case), three blot haemorrhages, a single cotton wool spot and fall in visual acuity which may be due to cataracts or maculopathy.

Background retinopathy (ie the presence of dot haemorrhages, blot haemorrhages and hard exudates) is common amongst diabetic patients and most will be referred to an ophthalmologist at some time. The significance of one cotton wool spot and three or more blot haemorrhages is that they indicate pre-proliferative changes; other such changes include venous bleeding and looping. Treatment is necessary to prevent proliferative changes developing which are the formation of new vessels. Proliferative retinopathy is an emergency, as vitreous haemorrhage, traction retinal detachment and blindness may occur.

3.33 Ventricular fibrillation   Answers: C D

Ventricular fibrillation produces bizarre QRS complexes. In a witnessed arrest precordial thump should be delivered, but otherwise it is a priority to deliver direct current (DC) shock immediately. Damage to the myocardium does occur with DC cardioversion, but the patient will die unless cardioversion is successful, therefore the patient should receive shocks until sinus rhythm is obtained. In persistent VF changing the paddle positions to a front back axis or using a different defibrillator may help. Ideally attempts to resuscitate should continue whilst the patient is still in VF although the length of time of resuscitation is a matter for clinical management. Ventricular fibrillation may be precipitated by ischaemic heart disease (eg MI), cardiomyopathy, or drugs (eg antiepileptics, tricyclic antidepressants and quinidine). These drugs predispose to ventricular arrhythmias in general, as well as to ventricular fibrillation. The prognosis for a patient in ventricular fibrillation is much better than for one in asystole.

3.34 Urinary tract infection   Answers: A B C D E

- A urinary tract infection is more likely to occur in women than men (women have a much shorter urethra and therefore less distance for bacteria to travel)
- Any instrumentation may introduce bacteria (eg catheterisation, cystoscopy)
- Stones in the renal tract form a nidus for bacteria, encouraging their growth
- Most congenital abnormalities (eg duplex systems) predispose to infections

General anaesthetic agents have an effect on the sacral nerve supply to the bladder predisposing to urinary retention; this allows bacteria to stay in the bladder longer, increasing the risk of infection.

3.35 Round face   Answers: A C E

This is an unusual question, but it does turn up occasionally. Hereditary factors may be responsible, and obesity and Cushing's syndrome are also causes. In nephrotic syndrome there may be such gross generalised oedema that the face appears round. Acromegaly will cause enlargement of the facial features but should not make the face particularly round. In some forms of muscular dystrophy, the facial muscles can be quite wasted and the face appears thin and drawn.

3.36 Nephrotic syndrome   **Answers: A C D**

Nephrotic syndrome is characterised by proteinuria of >3–5 g/24 h, hypoal-buminaemia and peripheral oedema. It is also associated with hypercholes-terolaemia.

Note the difference between the words 'characteristic' and 'diagnostic'. The latter implies that hypogammaglobulinaemia would only occur in nephrotic syndrome and no other medical condition, which is clearly not the case, but the term 'characteristic' is appropriate.

A hypercoagulable state is often associated with nephrotic syndrome and venous thrombosis is common.

Children have a better outcome because they tend to develop minimal change glomerulonephritis, which has the best prognosis, the condition often resolving completely.

The causes of nephrotic syndrome include glomerulonephritis (there are many subtypes, but the most important are minimal change, focal scle-rosing and membranous), diabetes, myeloma, SLE, infections such as malaria and drugs such as penicillamine and gold.

Treatment is supportive and diuretics should be used with salt-poor albumin, a high protein intake and treatment or prevention of intercurrent infection. The underlying cause should be sought and treated, and usually this involves a renal biopsy, but in children with highly selective proteinuria minimal change glomerulonephritis is highly likely and this can be treated with corticosteroids and cyclophosphamide in those who relapse.

Prognosis is good in children, when renal function is normal, and when hypertension is not present.

3.37 Pituitary ablation   **Answers: A C D**

In male patients, testosterone replacement is necessary, as the gonadotrophin hormones are no longer produced. Daily thyroxine replacement is necessary, as thyroid stimulating hormone (TSH) is no longer produced. Adrenocorticotropic hormone (ACTH) is absent and therefore hydrocortisone and prednisolone must be given daily. Note that mineralo-corticoid production by the adrenals is under the control of the renin–angiotensin axis and therefore does not need replacement. Antidiuretic hormone (ADH) loss necessitates desmopressin replacement.

Although growth hormone is produced by the anterior pituitary, in an adult it only has an effect on muscle mass and therefore is not replaced after pituitary ablation. Glucagon is produced by the pancreas and is not affected by the pituitary.

3.38 Hypertension

Answers: A B C D

A raised arterial blood pressure causes changes in the blood vessel wall. Plaques are more likely to develop and this increases the risk of embolic stroke. More important, however, is the risk of haemorrhagic stroke especially in hypertensive patients.

The increase in arterial pressure forces the heart to work harder, particularly the left ventricle, which has to pump against increased resistance. This increases the risk of left ventricular failure and the increased demand predisposes to myocardial infarction. Aortic stenosis is not associated with hypertension.

3.39 Rickets

Answers: A B D

Normal bone is composed of osteoid (bone matrix) which is mineralised. When there is normal bone, but it is reduced in mass per unit volume, osteopenia results. The combination of osteopenia and low-trauma fractures produces osteoporosis.

When bone is inadequately mineralised with calcium and phosphate, the bones become soft. This is usually caused by a defect in vitamin D availability or metabolism and produces rickets in children and osteomalacia in adults.

Vitamin D is necessary for the absorption of calcium and phosphate in the gut. A lack of vitamin D or an active metabolite therefore results in a low plasma calcium and low serum phosphate.

Parathyroid hormone levels rise as the serum calcium falls and the effect on bone is to increase osteoclastic resorption in an attempt to raise plasma calcium levels. It also promotes phosphate excretion via the kidneys, lowering the serum levels further. Serum alkaline phosphatase increases. Childhood rickets usually presents with bony deformity or failure of adequate growth. Clinical features include frontal bossing, bowing of the femur and tibia and an enlargement at the costochondral junction. The latter is termed 'rickety rosary'.

3.40 Arm swelling

Answers: A B C D

In general, swelling of the arm may be due to infection, inflammation, abnormal blood flow or abnormal lymphatic drainage. Venous obstruction can produce swelling distal to the obstruction and a clot in the axillary vein or subclavian vein may cause the whole arm to swell.

A blockage to lymphatic drainage occurs with lymph node infiltration with a tumour, or infection (eg lymphogranuloma). Removal of lymph nodes, for example as part of the treatment of breast surgery, or lymph node treatment with radiotherapy, will also produce lymphoedema. In patients who have had a stroke, disuse of the affected arm can also produce swelling.

Aortic dissection produces tearing interscapular pain, and unequal pulses and blood pressures between the two arms, but it will not cause swelling.

3.41 Asbestos exposure   Answers: B C D E

Asbestos exposure may produce no effect or cause asymptomatic plaques of the pleura, diaphragm or even the peritoneum. Asbestos exposure increases the risk of malignancy, both of the pleura (mesothelioma) and also the lung itself (bronchial carcinoma). The effects of asbestos on malignancy are synergistic with those of smoking. Lung fibrosis may occur, typically in the lower zone. Cardiac failure is not a typical complication unless there is severe lung damage sufficient to cause cor pulmonale and in any case this would lead to right heart failure rather than left ventricular failure.

3.42 Bone metastases   Answers: A B C

There are five important tumours that metastasise to bone and must be remembered: breast, bronchus, thyroid, kidney, prostate. Other tumours may also do this (eg melanoma), but the five mentioned above should be at the top of the list of differentials.

3.43 Weight loss   Answers: A D E

Considering the differential diagnosis of weight loss, it is important to consider functional (psychiatric) causes and medical causes.

Depression can certainly produce that level of weight loss, but anxiety on its own should not. Other causes such as anorexia nervosa must also be considered. Causes of weight loss include metabolic conditions, such as hypothyroidism and diabetes mellitus; malignancy; malabsorptive states and other gastrointestinal disorders, such as inflammatory bowel disease; and connective tissue disorders and chronic infections.

Bronchial adenomas are not malignant and another cause for weight loss should be suspected.

3.44 Weight gain   Answers: A C D

Weight gain may be due to an increase in muscle bulk, fat deposition or abnormal fluid retention. In nephrotic syndrome, hyperalbuminuria leads to oedema and weight gain. In pelvic malignancy, ascites often results, causing clinically significant weight gain. In congestive cardiac failure a low cardiac output stimulates the renin–angiotensin system resulting in secondary hyperaldosteronism which causes sodium and hence water retention. The weight gain with congestive cardiac failure may be considerable. Bronchial carcinoma produces significant weight loss and even with the hormone-secreting tumours which may produce substances such as ACTH, clinically significant weight gain is unlikely. Diabetes insipidus causes polyuria, poly-dipsia and weight loss.

3.45 Ankle jerk reflex   Answers: A B C D

An intact ankle jerk reflex depends on afferent sensory fibres from the soleus/gastrocnemius tendon, efferent motor fibres to the calf muscles, the calf muscles themselves and the neuromuscular junction. Damage at any of these sites will produce a reduced or absent reflex.

- Sensory fibres
  - These relay impulses from the stretch receptors in the tendon and enter the dorsal root in the spinal cord to form a reflex arc. Damage to the peripheral nerve may occur with diabetes mellitus and Guillain–Barré syndrome. Local S1 root lesions (eg tumour) may also occur. Dorsal column disease interrupts the pathway, for example syphilitic taboparesis, subacute combined degeneration of the cord.
- The efferent motor pathway
  - Anterior horn cell damage (eg polio).

Motor neurone disease may cause absent ankle jerks, but more commonly it causes upper motor neurone lesions and hence brisk reflexes.

Guillain–Barré syndrome also affects peripheral motor nerves as well as sensory nerves.

Myasthenia gravis affects the neuromuscular junction producing muscle weakness. There is characteristic fatigability of the reflexes, ie with repeated stimulation the reflex jerk becomes weaker (it is not usually absent).

Parkinson's disease should not affect the reflex jerks.

3.46 Bowing of the tibia
Answers: A C D

The important causes of bowing of the tibia include Paget's disease, rickets, syphilis or yaws, and polyosteotic fibrous dysplasia (Albright's disease).

3.47 Polyuria and polydipsia
Answers: A C E

Thirst and water regulation are largely controlled by ADH (vasopressin). Changes in plasma osmolarity are sensed by osmoreceptors in the hypothalamus and ADH secretion is altered. Disorders affecting this include inappropriate excess of the hormone (syndrome of inappropriate ADH), deficiency (eg diabetes insipidus), and organ resistance (eg nephrogenic diabetes insipidus). Hypokalaemia and hypercalcaemia damage the renal tubules producing nephrogenic diabetes insipidus. Water excretion is dependent on normal renal function. Acute renal failure tends to produce oliguria, whereas chronic renal failure produces polyuria.

Diabetes mellitus produces polyuria and polydipsia as the high sugar load exceeds the maximum re-absorptive capacity of the tubules and is excreted, taking water with it.

Hysteria is also a cause of polyuria and polydipsia.

3.48 Skin pigmentation
Answers: A C D

Pernicious anaemia may result in jaundice and this combined with the pallor of anaemia produces the characteristic lemon yellow tinge to the skin.

Haemochromatosis produces hyperpigmentation, which is generalised but more evident in sun-exposed areas. It is due to increased melanin secretion and may also occur in patients with primary biliary cirrhosis (jaundice is another reason for skin colour alteration in these patients).

Hypercarotinaemia causes a yellow discoloration of the skin that may be confused with jaundice. However, in the latter the sclera are typically involved, whereas in hypercarotinaemia the sclera are spared.

Carbon monoxide poisoning produces a pink coloration of the skin.

Lead poisoning tends to produce mucocutaneous discoloration rather than a generalised colour change.

You may be asked about Mongolian blue spot – the answer to this is false as it causes a local rather than generalised colour change.

3.49 Vomiting   Answers: A C D E

Vomiting may occur post-operatively, whatever the surgery performed, because general anaesthetic agents often cause gastroparesis.

Bowel obstruction, for example due to tumour, adhesions, strangulated hernia, etc, can produce vomiting (an early, predominant feature of proximal lesions), constipation (a predominant feature of distal, ie large bowel obstruction) and pain.

The vomiting centre in the brain receives afferents from the higher centres and from the gut and vestibular system and relays to the chemoreceptor trigger zone that stimulates vomiting. The chemoreceptor trigger zone also activated by drugs, for example opiates, dopaminergics, 5-HT and dopamine.

Acute labyrinthitis may cause vertigo and vomiting.

Ménière's disease causes vertigo, vomiting, tinnitus and deafness.

A low serum potassium is a consequence, not a cause, of vomiting.

3.50 Irritable bowel syndrome   Answers: All false

Irritable bowel syndrome usually causes abdominal pain that is often relieved by defaecation or the passage of wind. The patient may complain of constipation or diarrhoea, and a feeling of incomplete emptying of the rectum, but there is usually a fairly long history to this. Patients may also complain of being bloated and their clothes feeling too tight for them at the end of the day. It is more common in young people, especially women, and symptoms may be exacerbated by stress.

Weight loss, a change in bowel habit for the first time and blood per rectum are all serious symptoms which are not attributable to irritable bowel syndrome.

Improvement on a gluten-free diet suggests coeliac disease and dysphagia is a symptom of upper GI disease.

3.51 Investigations   Answer: C

Sarcoidosis should be diagnosed on history, examination (see Paper 1, Question 1.49) and investigations; abnormal investigations may include:

- Blood – hypercalcaemia, hypercalciuria, lymphopenia, occasionally eosinophilia; raised ESR, arterial blood gases may show a mild hypoxia

- Serum ACE – this is 2 SD above the normal mean value in over 75% of patients with untreated sarcoidosis
- Lung function tests – decreased lung volumes, reduced diffusing capacity (KCO); normal FEV_1/FVC ratio
- Radiology – lung fibrosis, hilar lymphadenopathy, reticulo-nodular shadowing; bone cysts may be present, particularly in the digits; MRI of neuro-sarcoid may show thickening of the meninges; gallium (not thallium) scanning may show increased uptake in the lungs
- Biopsy – transbronchial biopsy or lymph node biopsy is useful for pulmonary sarcoidosis where positive results occur in 90% even if there is no abnormality on chest X-ray; non-caseating granulomas are typical
- Kveim test – this is controversial as there is a risk of transmission of infection and it should be performed by specialists only.

Myocardial ischaemia may be apparent on an exercise ECG, but if the results are not conclusive, nuclear medicine investigations, such as thallium imaging, may be useful. The radioactive substance thallium-201 is given intravenously. It behaves like potassium and is taken up by healthy myocardium. Ischaemia or infarction therefore produces a cold spot where there is an absence of isotope. The isotope can be administered during exercise and an image taken shortly after. This is compared with the image obtained at rest; a cold spot on both scans indicates infarction, but a cold spot on the exercise scan that is not present on the resting scan indicates reversible ischaemia and may make coronary bypass surgery worthwhile.

A pyrophosphate scan may be used to identify acute myocardial infarction (1–5 days).

Left ventricular function can be assessed by echocardiography and by a multiple gated acquisition (MUGA) scan. The latter involves imaging the heart after administration of a radioisotope over many R–R intervals and a visible image of the heart through the whole cardiac cycle can be obtained as well as accurate measurements of ejection fraction, end diastolic volume, etc.

Lung metastases may be apparent on chest X-ray but are more clearly demonstrated on a CT image. At present, MRI is not routinely used for this. Caecal carcinoma is best imaged by use of a barium enema.

3.52 Hair

Answers: A B D E

Alopecia occurs when hair loss on the scalp is so extensive that it causes abnormal visibility of the scalp. It may be permanent, in which case the hair follicles have been damaged by scarring (eg lichen planus or discoid lupus erythematosus). If the follicles are intact, recovery may occur and hair loss is temporary (eg alopecia areata and some endocrine conditions).

Alopecia areata occurs in association with autoimmune diseases, such as thyrotoxicosis, Addison's disease, etc. Endocrine conditions include hyper-thyroidism, hypothyroidism and androgen overactivity in both males and females.

Other causes of reversible hair loss:

* drugs (eg lithium, vitamin A derivatives, chemotherapy, platinum derivatives)
* severe illness
* rapid weight loss
* iron deficiency
* stress
* after pregnancy.

Minoxidil and other drugs, such as cortisone and ciclosporin, cause hypertrichosis.

3.53 Screening

Answer: E

A good screening test must be sensitive and specific as well as feasible to use, ie low cost and acceptable to the patient.

Faecal occult blood testing can be useful in certain circumstances, for example to investigate a source of blood loss in anaemia, but it is not a good screening test for GI malignancy because the test is not specific enough. It is very sensitive (ie it will pick up even small amounts of blood) but common conditions such as haemorrhoids may give rise to a positive test producing a lack of specificity for GI tumours.

Cortisol levels fluctuate considerably during the day and are raised in obesity and with stress. Of more use is a 24-h collection of urine for cortisol or measurement of cortisol after dexamethasone suppression.

A resting ECG is most unlikely to show asymptomatic cardiac ischaemia. CA125 is very good screening test for ovarian carcinoma because it is both sensitive and specific. Genetic testing is not a good screening test for breast cancer. Although much media attention has been devoted to the two oncogenes BRCA1 and BRCA2, most people with breast cancer do not have these genes and furthermore having these genes does not guarantee the development of breast cancer. As the only prophylactic measure for breast cancer is bilateral mastectomy, any test must be much more specific and sensitive.

3.54 Epidemiology

Answers: B C

The prevalence of a disease is the number of cases suffering from the disease per head of the population at any time. The prevalence of a disease is determined by a cross-sectional study of the population.

The incidence of a disease is the number of new cases diagnosed per head of the population in a given time, usually a year. It is determined using a longitudinal study.

If an illness is long lasting (eg Crohn's disease or asthma), there will be more people with the disease at a given time than if the disease were short lived (eg malignant brain tumour). Prevalence therefore depends on the duration of illness.

For conditions with a high case fatality, ie a large number of those with the disease die, then the mortality rate can be used to estimate the incidence of the disease.

The prevalence of asthma is 5–15% of the population and is higher in the second decade of life.

3.55 Iron

Answers: A B

A low serum iron occurs in iron deficiency anaemia, anaemia of chronic disease and malignancy. Rheumatoid arthritis causes iron deficiency for many reasons, for example iron deficiency secondary to GI bleeds from non-steroidal treatment, megaloblastic anaemia/pancytopenia from methotrexate therapy, neutropenia from Felty's syndrome and the anaemia of chronic disease.

The total iron binding capacity (TIBC) is raised in iron deficiency anaemia but reduced in chronic disease or malignancy.

3.56 Faecal fat

Answers: B D E

Fat in the diet is mainly in the form of triglycerides. These are emulsified in the stomach and then hydrolysed by pancreatic lipases. Mixed micelles are formed and chylomicrons are absorbed into the lymphatics. Bile salts are synthesised by the liver, stored in the gallbladder and enter the duodenum.

They aggregate with the fat to form the micelles. Bile salts are reabsorbed in the terminal ileum and transported back to the liver (enterohepatic circulation).

It can be deduced that interruption of these processes may result in fat malabsorption.

- Bile salts
  Liver disease; obstructive jaundice results in decreased bile salt production
  Crohn's disease damages the terminal ileum, the site of bile salt reabsorption
  Deconjugation of bile salts due to bacterial overgrowth renders bile salts ineffective
- Pancreatic enzymes
  For example, chronic pancreatitis; raised gastrin levels in Zollinger–Ellison syndrome cause increased gastric acid production which reduces the intestinal pH and inhibits the pancreatic enzymes which require an alkaline medium
- Area for fat absorption
  For example, coeliac disease, tropical sprue, intestinal resection.

3.57 Pleural effusion   Answers: B C D

Oesophageal rupture causes a mediastinitis and pleural effusion; oesophagitis does not. The effusion is an exudate. Tuberculous effusions have a high protein content (exudate) and low sugar, and may contain acid-fast bacilli. Aspiration of an effusion to obtain acid-fast bacilli should be preceded by pleural biopsy as this increases the yield of bacilli. Rheumatoid arthritis can produce several changes in the lung: nodules which may cavitate, pleural effusions and lung fibrosis. Any cardiothoracic surgery, such as for valve replacement, bypass grafting or lung resection, often causes a pleural effusion.

3.58 Generalised lymphadenopathy   Answers: A C E

See Paper 2, explanation 2.32. Other options that have been reported include rubella (true) and Still's disease (true).

3.59 Death certificates   Answers: B D E

The important observations that need to be made before certifying death are:

- absence of response to external stimuli
- absence of a central pulse which must be felt for 1 min
- absence of heart sounds for at least 1 min
- absence of breath sounds for at least 1 min
- both pupils must be non-reactive to light and must be fixed and dilated.

The JVP is irrelevant and the radial pulse is not important as it is not a central pulse.

3.60 Angina   Answers: A B C D

Angina may be precipitated by anaemia; this causes an increase in workload of the heart.

Thyroxine causes an increase in heart rate and cardiac output, and stress or emotion may provoke angina. Eating a large meal may increase the workload of the heart.

Myocardial infarction may actually cure angina. This is because ischaemia is painful but if that area dies due to infarction, it will no longer produce pain.

BEST OF FIVE AND MULTIPLE CHOICE QUESTIONS PAPER 4

60 questions: time allowed 2½ hours

Best of Five Questions
Mark your answers with a tick (True) in the box provided.

4.1 A 45-year-old lady with previous rheumatic fever and mitral valve replacement (on warfarin) is admitted at the request of her GP with an INR of 7.3. She has no direct complaints. Urinalysis +++ blood. What is the correct course of action?

- ❑ A Administer 2 packs of fresh frozen plasma
- ❑ B Give vitamin K 0.5 mg IV
- ❑ C Stop warfarin
- ❑ D Give protamine 2 mg IV
- ❑ E Halve regular dose of warfarin

4.2 A 48-year-old man is admitted with chronic alcoholic liver disease. He gives little history himself. On examination: grade 1 encephalopathy, 4-cm hepar and significant ascites. Which ONE of the following is most reflective of synthetic liver function?

- ❑ A Prothrombin time and ALP
- ❑ B Prothrombin time and albumin
- ❑ C ALP and AST
- ❑ D Albumin and ALP
- ❑ E Prothrombin time, albumin and ALP

4.3 A 32-year-old women attends casualty acutely short of breath with right-sided pleuritic chest discomfort and dizziness. On examination: no chest wall tenderness, nil adventitious sounds on auscultation. Calves unremarkable. ECG – sinus tachycardia 128 bpm. D-Dimer 0.79 mg/l. Oxygen saturation 91% on room air. VQ scan was reported as low probability for a pulmonary embolus. What is the most appropriate next step?

❏ A   Investigations complete; the patient may be discharged
❏ B   Undertake bronchoscopy
❏ C   Repeat VQ scan the following day
❏ D   Treat as for a lower respiratory tract infection (LRTI)
❏ E   Request a CT pulmonary angiogram

4.4   **An 18-year-old university student complains of a short history of headache of gradual onset associated with malaise. On examination: temperature 37.8°C, no focal neurology. CT brain – normal. Lumbar puncture was performed: clear, opening pressure 15 mmH$_2$O, no organisms seen, total protein 0.91 g/l, RCC 1/mm^3, WCC 154/mm^3 (>95% lymphocytes). What diagnosis does this most likely indicate?**

❏ A   Idiopathic intracranial hypertension
❏ B   Viral meningitis
❏ C   Tuberculous meningitis
❏ D   Cerebral abscess
❏ E   Bacterial meningitis

4.5   **A 22-year-old asthmatic reaches casualty acutely short of breath, unable to speak in complete sentences, tachypneic and with a tachycardia of 122 bpm. On examination: severe inspiratory wheeze. She receives nebulised salbutamol and ipratropium bromide. IV hydrocortisone administered. At the time of the arterial blood gas shown below she had been on an IV salbutamol infusion for 45 min. ABG (on 10 l via mask): pH 7.50, PO_2 10.3 kPa, PCO_2 5.6 kPa, HCO$_3^-$ 28.4 mmol/l. What is the next most appropriate course of action?**

❏ A   Start CPAP
❏ B   Start NIPPV
❏ C   Start an aminophylline infusion
❏ D   Administer oral magnesium
❏ E   Request anaesthetic assessment for ICU

4.6   **A 36-year-old telephonist with a 5-year history of sarcoidosis admits to increasing shortness of breath over the past 4 weeks when attending respiratory outpatients. This is his fourth episode of this nature since his diagnosis. He has previously responded well to tapered doses of oral steroids. What initial test would be most helpful before prescribing steroids to assess his current pulmonary status objectively?**

❏ A CXR
❏ B Pulmonary function tests with transfer factor
❏ C ABG
❏ D Serum ACE level
❏ E High-resolution computed tomography (HRCT) of chest

4.7 **A 62-year-old gentleman with long-standing multiple sclerosis (MS) is admitted due to increasing problems with his care in the community. He is bed-bound with a spastic paraparesis. He is noted to have a permanent 14-gauge urinary catheter in situ. The family informs the nursing staff this has not been changed for some time. Your senior colleague wishes for the catheter to be replaced. Which one of the following statements is most accurate?**

❏ A The catheter should be increased from a 14 to a 16 gauge when replaced
❏ B Given the paraparesis local anaesthetic gel is not essential
❏ C A male chaperone is required
❏ D A single dose of prophylactic gentamicin is advisable
❏ E The catheter will need replacing again in 9 months time

4.8 **A 17-year-old girl takes 45 of her step-father's aspirin tablets following an argument with her boyfriend. Twelve hours into her admission the following ABG and biochemistry tests were performed. pH 7.27, PCO_2 3.0 kPa, PO_2 14.3 kPa, HCO_3^- 16.2 mmol/l, BE –7.4 mmol/l. Na^+ 143 mmol/l, K^+ 4.5 mmol/l, Cl^- 107 mmol/l, urea 12.4 mmol/l, creatinine 87 μmol/l. What is the patient's anion gap?**

❏ A 24.3 mmol/l
❏ B 21.3 mmol/l
❏ C 20.1 mmol/l
❏ D 47.7 mmol/l
❏ E 2.13 mmol/l

4.9 A 53-year-old lady with bipolar affective disorder is brought to casualty by her son after being found at home with two empty bottles of her prescribed medication (lithium) by her side. She is believed to have taken the tablets several hours ago. No other tablets were found at the scene. On examination – global hyper-reflexia. Her serum lithium level is 5.9 mmol/l. Hb 12.3 g/dl, WCC 9.1 × 10⁹/l, Plts 199 × 10⁹/l. Na⁺ 136 mmol/l, K⁺ 5.0 mmol/l, urea 28 mmol/l, Cr 550 μmol/l. Which one of the following is the treatment of choice?

☐ A Oral charcoal
☐ B Aim fluid balance: Input = Output + 1000 ml
☐ C Set up IV infusion of frusemide
☐ D Commence haemodialysis
☐ E Commence IVI of human immunoglobulin (IgG)

4.10 A 35-year-old teacher complains of lethargy and generalised aches and pains, especially in the shoulders and hands. She has been on sick leave from school for the past 4 months. The GP letter indicates a history of irritable bowel syndrome. He also states that he tried a short course of steroids and anti-inflammatory medication with no effect. On examination: multiple tender points in various muscle groups. No discernible joint disease. What is the likely diagnosis?

☐ A Polymyalgia
☐ B Polymyositis
☐ C Hypothyroidism
☐ D Fibromyalgia
☐ E Systemic lupus erythematosus

4.11 A 69-year-old residential home dweller is admitted with acute-onset severe abdominal pain associated with bloody diarrhoea. She has a history of angina, chronic obstructive pulmonary disease (COPD) and atrial fibrillation. Her drugs include a statin, beta-blocker and digoxin. Erect CXR: no free air. Which one of the following diagnoses is most likely?

☐ A Pseudomembranous colitis
☐ B Infective diarrhoea
☐ C Colorectal carcinoma
☐ D Ischaemic colitis
☐ E Angiodysplasia

4.12 A 36-year-old teacher attends the thyroid clinic with a 4-month history of a swelling within the neck accompanied by weight loss of 5 kg. On examination: thin, hands sweaty to touch. Diffuse smooth swelling of the thyroid gland. She is in atrial fibrillation. Lid lag is noted and proximal myopathy is observed. A rash is seen over the anterior aspects of the legs in keeping with pretibial myxoedema. Which clinical sign is most suggestive of Grave's disease as the cause of her clinical hyperthyroidism?

- ❏ A Diffuse thyroid swelling
- ❏ B Lid retraction
- ❏ C Pretibial myxoedema
- ❏ D Atrial fibrillation
- ❏ E Proximal myopathy

4.13 A 34-year-old schizophrenic has been known to the mental health services for several years with a remitting and relapsing course of disease. His consultant, in conjunction with the patient's community psychiatric nurse (CPN), decides to commence clozapine. As part of the prescription he is enrolled into the Clozapine Monitoring Service programme. Which one of the following statements most accurately reflects the main reason for enrolment?

- ❏ A Due to a limited budget for this medication
- ❏ B To monitor the white cell count
- ❏ C To monitor liver function tests
- ❏ D To allow audit of the drug to be recorded
- ❏ E To monitor renal function

4.14 A 24-year-old known epileptic patient complains of a 4-day history of unsteadiness and altered vision. Colleagues have commented that he appears drunk whilst at work. He attended neurology outpatients 3 weeks previously. On examination: wide-based gait, past pointing and intention tremor. Which one of the following medications is likely to be responsible?

- ❏ A Phenytoin
- ❏ B Sodium valproate
- ❏ C Carbamazepine
- ❏ D Atenolol
- ❏ E Gabapentin

4.15   You are asked to see a 45-year-old woman who says her mood has been 'rubbish' for months. She complains of episodes lasting around 5 min where she is suddenly very anxious, hyperventilates and feels nauseous whilst thinking she is going to die from a heart attack. On direct questioning you find that over the last 2 months she has lost interest in ballroom dancing and going to the cinema, which she previously enjoyed. She has also been so tired she has missed several days at work. Things have got even worse in the last month with these episodes of anxiety happening at least once a week and sometimes she even wishes she wasn't alive, although she says she would never do anything to harm herself. There is no physical abnormality. What is her most likely diagnosis?

❑   A   Generalised anxiety disorder
❑   B   Panic disorder
❑   C   Depression with secondary panic attacks
❑   D   Agoraphobia
❑   E   Chronic fatigue syndrome

Multiple Choice Questions

Mark your answers with a tick (True) or a cross (False) in the box provided. Leave the box blank for 'Don't know'. Do not look at the answers until you have completed the whole question paper.

4.16 Concerning acute deep venous thrombosis

- ❏ A About 20% embolise to the lung
- ❏ B The first-line radiological investigation is a venogram
- ❏ C Admission is required until warfarin treatment is established
- ❏ D An above-knee deep venous thrombosis requires 3 months of anticoagulation
- ❏ E A below-knee deep venous thrombosis is of no clinical significance

4.17 Pulmonary embolism is unlikely if the

- ❏ A Partial pressure of oxygen is >10.7 kPa
- ❏ B Chest X-ray is normal
- ❏ C D-Dimer is <3 ml/l
- ❏ D Respiratory rate is <20 respirations per minute
- ❏ E Patient is below 30 years of age

4.18 In the assessment of an acute asthma attack

- ❏ A A peak flow less than 50% best predicted is an indication of a severe attack
- ❏ B Hypertension indicates a life-threatening attack
- ❏ C Tachycardia >110 bpm indicates a severe attack
- ❏ D A PCO_2 <2.5 kPa indicates a need for ventilation
- ❏ E Absence of wheeze indicates the attack is mild

4.19 A patient with hypertension requires admission to hospital if

- ❏ A The diastolic blood pressure is >130 mmHg
- ❏ B Blood pressure is known to have risen suddenly
- ❏ C Papilloedema is present
- ❏ D Seizures occur
- ❏ E There is co-existent diabetes

4.20   The following ECG changes are diagnostic of acute myocardial infarction:

❏   A   ST elevation of greater than or equal to 1 mm in leads AVR and AVL
❏   B   ST elevation of greater than or equal to 1 mm in leads AVL and III
❏   C   ST elevation of greater than or equal to 1 mm in leads V3 and V4
❏   D   ST elevation of greater than or equal to 2 mm in leads V5 and V6
❏   E   New right bundle branch block (RBBB)

4.21   The following are contraindications to thrombolysis

❏   A   Aortic dissection
❏   B   Menstruation
❏   C   Previous TB infection
❏   D   Previous subarachnoid haemorrhage
❏   E   Liver biopsy 1 month ago

4.22   Regarding an abdominal X-ray

❏   A   The small bowel is centrally placed
❏   B   The large bowel does not normally contain gas
❏   C   The small bowel is dilated if it is >3 cm in diameter
❏   D   The large bowel is dilated if it is >5.5 cm in diameter
❏   E   The large bowel has folds called valvulae conniventes

4.23   In a patient with unstable angina

❏   A   There is an increased risk of myocardial infarction
❏   B   Hospital admission is sometimes necessary
❏   C   Troponin levels rarely alter management
❏   D   Warfarin treatment should be started
❏   E   A beta-agonist should be given intravenously

4.24   A patient with a gastrointestinal bleed is deemed to be at high risk if

❏   A   The haemoglobin is <10 g/dl
❏   B   Is over 50 years of age
❏   C   The pulse rate is >100 bpm
❏   D   There is fresh melaena
❏   E   There is a postural drop in diastolic blood pressure

4.25   In the treatment of acute asthma

- ❏ A   Low-concentration oxygen should be given initially
- ❏ B   Intravenous salbutamol should be started if a nebuliser has failed to produce improvement
- ❏ C   Nebulised ipratropium bromide helps most patients
- ❏ D   Nebulised magnesium may help
- ❏ E   Fluid restriction to prevent pulmonary oedema is often necessary

4.26   Regarding the JVP

- ❏ A   Cannon waves occur in tricuspid stenosis
- ❏ B   It is raised in left ventricular failure
- ❏ C   It falls on inspiration
- ❏ D   It is raised in cardiac tamponade
- ❏ E   Large V waves will occur in mitral regurgitation

4.27   Cerebellar lesions cause the following

- ❏ A   An increase in tone
- ❏ B   Extensor plantar response
- ❏ C   Ipsilateral neurological signs
- ❏ D   Slurred speech
- ❏ E   Resting tremor

4.28   Which of the following conditions are associated with gut malignancy?

- ❏ A   Familial adenomatous polyposis coli
- ❏ B   *Helicobacter pylori*
- ❏ C   Coeliac disease
- ❏ D   Iron deficiency anaemia
- ❏ E   Reflux oesophagitis

4.29   Benign intracranial hypertension

- ❏ A   Is more common in women
- ❏ B   Is associated with certain drugs
- ❏ C   Causes papilloedema only if associated with a tumour
- ❏ D   Is treated by repeated lumbar puncture
- ❏ E   Is characterised by frequent headaches

4.30   Causes of gynaecomastia include

❏ A   Ranitidine
❏ B   Testicular tumours
❏ C   Liver failure
❏ D   Hyperprolactinaemia
❏ E   Cyproterone

4.31   Hypoglycaemia may be caused by

❏ A   Diabetic ketoacidosis
❏ B   Aspirin
❏ C   Alcohol
❏ D   Carcinoid
❏ E   Sepsis

4.32   Acute stroke and transient ischaemia attacks

❏ A   A transient ischaemic attack often resolves within 48 h
❏ B   All patients with a stroke should have a CT scan or an MRI
❏ C   All patients with a stroke should have an echocardiogram
❏ D   All patients with a stroke should have an ECG
❏ E   All patients with a stroke should have a carotid duplex study

4.33   Intracranial haemorrhage

❏ A   Cerebellar haemorrhage requires neurosurgical referral
❏ B   10% of CT scans appear normal in the presence of a subarachnoid haemorrhage
❏ C   Subdural haemorrhage is usually venous in nature
❏ D   Extradural haemorrhage has a bi-concave or lentiform appearance
❏ E   Intracerebral haemorrhage is often due to hypertension

4.34   Status epilepticus is

❏ A   A continuous generalised tonic clonic seizure
❏ B   Any seizure lasting more than 3 min
❏ C   More than two discrete seizures with incomplete recovery between them
❏ D   New-onset epilepsy
❏ E   Fits occurring despite treatment

4.35   Activated charcoal reduces drug absorption of

- ❏   A   Ferrous sulphate
- ❏   B   Lithium
- ❏   C   Phenytoin
- ❏   D   Digoxin
- ❏   E   Aspirin

4.36   Causes of a resting tremor include

- ❏   A   Parkinson's disease
- ❏   B   Anxiety
- ❏   C   Cerebellar disorders
- ❏   D   Alcohol withdrawal
- ❏   E   Hypothyroidism

4.37   A man of 25 years has a swollen painful knee, a prolonged partial thromboplastin time and a normal prothrombin time. The differential diagnosis includes

- ❏   A   Temporal arteritis
- ❏   B   Christmas disease
- ❏   C   Haemophilia A
- ❏   D   Factor VII deficiency
- ❏   E   Von Willebrand's disease

4.38   Randomised controlled clinical trials

- ❏   A   Are the only convincing method of demonstrating efficacy of a drug
- ❏   B   Require a cross-over period
- ❏   C   Should be done retrospectively
- ❏   D   Are ideally double-blind
- ❏   E   Need approximately 100 subjects to detect a drug side-effect

4.39   The following are complications of IV drug abuse

- ❏   A   Endocarditis
- ❏   B   Tetanus
- ❏   C   Cerebral abscess
- ❏   D   Pulmonary embolism
- ❏   E   Hepatitis A

4.40   Sickle cell anaemia is often associated with

❑   A   Defective urinary concentrating ability
❑   B   Increased risk of osteomyelitis
❑   C   Anaemia at birth
❑   D   Swollen painful hands in toddlers
❑   E   Enlarged spleen

4.41 Features consistent with a diagnosis of mitral stenosis include

❑   A   A third heart sound
❑   B   An opening snap just after the second heart sound
❑   C   Displaced apex beat
❑   D   Early diastolic murmur with presystolic accentuation
❑   E   Atrial fibrillation

4.42   The following refer to the insertion of an intercostal chest drain

❑   A   The drain tip should point upwards for a pleural effusion
❑   B   The drain tip should point downwards for a pneumothorax
❑   C   The use of a trocar is advised
❑   D   An effusion is best drained with a long small-bore tube
❑   E   The ideal position is the 7th intercostal space, mid-clavicular line

4.43   Causes of haemoptysis include

❑   A   Cystic fibrosis
❑   B   Goodpasture's syndrome
❑   C   Lung fibrosis
❑   D   Tuberculosis
❑   E   Left ventricular failure

4.44   The following are contraindications to renal biopsy

❑   A   Uncooperative patient
❑   B   Small kidneys
❑   C   Coagulation defect
❑   D   Single (non-transplanted) kidney
❑   E   Previous renal biopsy

4.45   The following skin conditions are associated with malignancy

- ❏ A   Dermatomyositis
- ❏ B   Acanthosis nigricans
- ❏ C   Chronic eczema
- ❏ D   Psoriasis
- ❏ E   Mycosis fungoides

4.46   Diabetic patients

- ❏ A   Need to inform the DVLA of their condition
- ❏ B   Should be given human insulin in preference to porcine insulin
- ❏ C   Can now be given insulin orally, avoiding the need for injections
- ❏ D   Should stop taking metformin when having an intravenous urogram
- ❏ E   Should stop their insulin if they are too ill to eat

4.47   High-dose oxygen treatment is advised for a patient with

- ❏ A   Acute asthma and a PCO_2 of 3 kPa
- ❏ B   Acute asthma and a PCO_2 of 6.5 kPa
- ❏ C   Chronic obstructive pulmonary disease
- ❏ D   Pneumonia
- ❏ E   Pulmonary embolism

4.48   The following are true of lipid-lowering drugs

- ❏ A   The aim of treatment is to raise LDL and lower HDL cholesterol
- ❏ B   They are only effective in secondary prevention of coronary heart disease
- ❏ C   Statins are used to treat hypercholesterolaemia
- ❏ D   Fibrates are used to treat hypertriglyceridaemia
- ❏ E   Fibrates are used to treat mixed hyperlipidaemia

4.49   Primary tumours which commonly metastasise to the lung include

- ❏ A   Breast
- ❏ B   Brain
- ❏ C   Thyroid
- ❏ D   Kidney
- ❏ E   Prostate

4.50   Infective causes of colitis include

❑ A   Tapeworm infection
❑ B   Salmonella
❑ C   Influenza
❑ D   *E. coli*
❑ E   *Clostridium difficile*

4.51   The following are true of audit studies

❑ A   They are the same as research
❑ B   Large sample sizes are essential
❑ C   They are observational
❑ D   They are susceptible to bias
❑ E   Statistical analysis cannot be performed

4.52   A diabetic patient has an autonomic neuropathy. As a result he may suffer from the following

❑ A   Nocturnal diarrhoea
❑ B   Postural hypotension
❑ C   Impotence
❑ D   Urine retention
❑ E   Increased sweating

4.53   Causes of Horner's syndrome include

❑ A   Herpes zoster infection
❑ B   Stroke
❑ C   Carotid dissection
❑ D   Lung carcinoma
❑ E   Trauma to the neck

4.54   Investigations which are useful in the diagnosis of myasthenia gravis include

❑ A   Epsilon test
❑ B   Anticholinesterase antibodies
❑ C   Electromyogram (EMG)
❑ D   Chest X-ray
❑ E   CT scan of the brain

4.55   Causes of cataract include

- ❑ A   Increase in age
- ❑ B   Diabetes mellitus
- ❑ C   Glaucoma
- ❑ D   Trauma
- ❑ E   Prolonged contact lens use

4.56   The following apply to the normal ECG

- ❑ A   It is recorded using 12 electrodes
- ❑ B   V4 and V5 record from the interventricular septum
- ❑ C   The normal axis is –30 to +90
- ❑ D   Down-sloping ST depression is a non-specific finding
- ❑ E   The PR interval is recorded from the start of the P wave to the R wave peak

4.57   The following are signs of a parietal lobe lesion

- ❑ A   Grasp reflex
- ❑ B   Emotional lability
- ❑ C   Homonymous quadrantanopia
- ❑ D   Sensory inattention
- ❑ E   Difficulty calculating numbers

4.58   Pulmonary fibrosis is a recognised sequel to

- ❑ A   Sarcoidosis
- ❑ B   Rheumatoid arthritis
- ❑ C   Radiotherapy
- ❑ D   Asbestosis
- ❑ E   Emphysema

4.59   Features of multiple myeloma include

- ❑ A   Fractures
- ❑ B   Hypercalcaemia
- ❑ C   Renal failure
- ❑ D   Raised alkaline phosphatase
- ❑ E   Hypogammaglobulinaemia

4.60   **Raynaud's phenomenon is a recognised feature of**

❏   A   Cryoglobulinaemia
❏   B   Scleroderma
❏   C   Diabetes mellitus
❏   D   Cervical rib
❏   E   Buerger's disease

─────────────── **END** ───────────────

**Go over your answers until your time is up. Correct answers
and teaching notes are overleaf**

BEST OF FIVE AND MULTIPLE CHOICE QUESTIONS PAPER 4
Answers

The correct answer options for each question are given below.

4.1	C	4.31	B C D E
4.2	B	4.32	B D
4.3	E	4.33	A C D E
4.4	B	4.34	A C
4.5	E	4.35	C D E
4.6	B	4.36	A B D
4.7	D	4.37	B C
4.8	A	4.38	D
4.9	D	4.39	A B C D
4.10	D	4.40	A B D
4.11	D	4.41	B E
4.12	C	4.42	All false
4.13	B	4.43	A B D E
4.14	A	4.44	A B C D
4.15	C	4.45	A B E
4.16	All false	4.46	A D
4.17	A D	4.47	A B D E
4.18	A C	4.48	C D E
4.19	A B C D	4.49	A C D
4.20	D	4.50	B D E
4.21	A D	4.51	C D
4.22	A C D	4.52	A B C D
4.23	A	4.53	B C D E
4.24	A C D E	4.54	C D
4.25	All false	4.55	A B C D
4.26	C D	4.56	C
4.27	C D	4.57	C D E
4.28	A B C D	4.58	A B C D
4.29	A B D E	4.59	A B C D
4.30	B C	4.60	A B D

BEST OF FIVE AND MULTIPLE CHOICE QUESTIONS PAPER 4
Answers and Teaching Notes

4.1 C: Stop warfarin

Warfarin is a commonly prescribed but also a potentially life-threatening drug when poorly controlled. It is the most popular oral anticoagulant, antagonising the effect of vitamin K. It has a wide range of indications, the commonest being in atrial fibrillation (with embolism risk), the treatment of deep venous thrombosis/pulmonary embolism (DVT/PE) and in those with mechanical prosthetic heart valves. The INR (an indicator of the prothrombin time) varies depending on its indication for use.

Indication for use	INR
DVT, PE, AF, rheumatic mitral valve disease	2.0–2.5
Recurrent DVT/PE, mechanical prosthetic valves	3.0–3.5

All the above options are potentially correct courses of action in different coagulopathies. The INR, along with the clinical status of the patient, guide the management choice.

INR/Bleeding status	Action
Major bleeding	Stop warfarin AND give vitamin K 5 mg IV OR fresh frozen plasma 15 ml/kg
INR > 6.0 WITH no/minor bleeding	Stop warfarin and restart when INR < 5.0. If other risk factors for bleeding given vitamin K 0.5 mg
INR <6.0 BUT >0.5 above target INR	Stop warfarin or reduce dose until INR <5.0

In this case therefore the correct treatment would be stop the warfarin and restart after the INR is less than 5.0. Overzealous correction in the absence of major bleeding when a prosthetic valve is in situ may cause further problems.

4.2 B: Prothrombin time and albumin

Liver function tests give an important insight into the nature of any liver impairment. Broadly speaking ALT and AST represent parenchymal function, ALP and GGT reflect obstructive disease and perhaps most importantly albumin and prothrombin time indicate the synthetic ability of the liver. The liver can sustain significant insults, both chronic and acute, and recover full function, such is its powers of regeneration. Its role of protein synthesis – reflected in serum blood tests by albumin – is an important indicator of 'liver health'. Likewise as the liver synthesises vitamin K when its functional capacity is impaired this will manifest as a prolonged pro-thrombin time. In acute liver failure these markers of synthetic function are hugely important in the overall assessment of the requirement for liver transplant.

4.3 E: Request a CT pulmonary angiogram

Pulmonary embolus and its investigation is an everyday medical issue. Imaging holds the key in making a definitive diagnosis and so triggering the commencement of anticoagulation therapy. Clinical suspicion may be high and supported by the findings of preliminary investigations. A sinus tachycardia on ECG, a low PaO_2 on arterial blood gas (ABG) and a raised D-dimer all raise clinical suspicions but are insufficient in isolation.

In most circumstances VQ (ventilation–perfusion) imaging is undertaken first although this is changing with the greater readability of multi-slice CT. This nuclear imaging scan will demonstrate a mismatched defect between ventilation and perfusion if a pulmonary embolus is present. The area of lung is ventilated, but not adequately perfused – the mismatch. Reports can be given as low, intermediate and high probability. Low probability still confers a risk of up to 15%. Therefore, if clinical suspicion is high – as is the case from this clinical scenario – further imaging should be requested. Previously this meant catheter pulmonary angiography, however with the advent of fast multi-slice CT this may now be done using computed tomography pulmonary angiography (CTPA). An embolus is seen as a 'filling defect' (an area which is not filled with contrast within the vessel).

4.4 B: Viral meningitis

Headache is a common complaint and a popular cause for medical admission is the onset of an acute headache. Two major diagnoses raise concern, especially in the young and previously well: subarachnoid haemorrhage (SAH) and bacterial meningitis. Both are potentially life threatening if not acted upon speedily. Those in institutional environments, such as schools and university accommodation, are particularly susceptible to infectious causes.

CT brain imaging may be normal in both bacterial meningitis and SAH in which case examination of the cerebrospinal fluid offers the diagnostic key.

The significant findings on lumbar puncture are a raised total protein and a mild to moderately elevated white cell count. The differential white cell count narrows the differential diagnoses. A 95% lymphocyte predominance excludes bacterial meningitis and cerebral abscess, unless partially treated. This scenario does not suggest any antibiotics have been administered. Both viral and tuberculous meningitis potentially give this CSF picture but the most likely would be a viral origin.

4.5 E: Request anaesthetic assessment for ICU

An acute asthma attack is one of the key medical emergencies. Detailed knowledge is essential and acute medical emergencies frequently appear in final exams. The guidelines for treatment are outlined and regularly updated by the British Thoracic Society and feature in each edition of the *British National Formulary* (BNF).

Two key learning points may be extracted from this question. Firstly, informing the anaesthetic team of a 'sick' asthmatic patient is essential, as rapid intubation may be required.

Features of a life-threatening attack.

- Cyanosis
- Silent chest
- Poor respiratory effort* or exhaustion
- Peak flow < 33% normal
- Agitation, confusion or altered conscious level
- Hypotension

Secondly, a normal or high PCO_2 on an ABG is a very worrying sign in an acute asthmatic – not least one who has received a significant amount of treatment with a poor response. Given the tachypnoea which accompanies an attack, CO_2 is 'blown off' and should give a respiratory alkalosis. A normal or raised CO_2 therefore indicates a tired* asthmatic who is likely to require assisted ventilation. This patient has reached the end of the line of ward-based treatment and requires a period of supportive therapy in the form of ventilation in ICU.

Treatment of acute asthma

High-flow oxygen
Salbutamol ± ipratropium bromide nebulisers
IV hydrocortisone
±IV infusion salbutamol (or aminophylline)
±IV magnesium (*evidence still soft*)
ICU (intubation and mechanical ventilation)

4.6 B: Pulmonary function tests with transfer factor

Sarcoidosis is a systematic idiopathic disease most frequently seen in clinical practice with respiratory manifestations. Respiratory sarcoidosis may be divided into four categories radiologically:

1. Hilar and mediastinal node involvement
2. Nodal and parenchymal involvement
3. Parenchymal involvement
4. Pulmonary fibrosis.

Lung disease is often very sensitive to steroids and during an exacerbation courses of high-dose tapered prednisolone are prescribed. The pulmonary function picture is typically a restrictive pattern (interstitial fibrosis is the underlying pathological process) with a reduced transfer factor. The level of transfer factor is sensitive to exacerbations and treatment of the disease. HRCT is equally important in establishing the degree and nature of inter-stitial disease and may be performed with disease progression. However, it would not be the initial test and given the radiation dose involved unlikely to be performed on every occasion the patient complains of worsening of their symptoms. Serum ACE has some value if elevated in observing a reduction in levels with treatment but is insufficient in isolation.

4.7 D: A single dose of prophylactic gentamicin is advisable

Permanent indwelling urinary catheters are often used but not without problems. It is essential if a decision is made for a permanent catheter (be it urethral or suprapubic) to be sited that measures are in place for its regular routine replacement. It is a foreign body and a portal of entry for infection. Urinary sepsis in this type of patient can be devastating and fatal. A chaperone is essential – the sex is not an issue as long as the patient has been given a choice. Given the aseptic requirements of placing a catheter an assistant is required (for example a nurse) who can serve also as the chaperone. It is not a routine procedure to change the size on replacement. However, it is vital that for *re-catheterisation* a single (stat) dose of gentamicin is considered and, unless there is good reason (eg significant renal impairment), administered before the catheter is replaced. This is prophylaxis against introducing infection whilst changing the catheter.

4.8. A: 24.3 mmol/l

Aspirin is a salicylate, which is acidic in nature. When ingested in excess, as in a deliberate overdose, a metabolic acidosis occurs. A salicylate overdose causes an anion gap metabolic acidosis. If the anion gap is increased it is due to the presence of an exogenous acid or acids normally present in unmeasured small quantities. This is calculated by subtracting the main anions (negative charge) in the plasma, bicarbonate and chloride, from the main cations (positive charge), sodium and potassium. The anion gap is usually composed of negatively charged proteins, organic acids and phosphate.

Calculation of anion gap = $(Na^+ + K^+) - (HCO_3^- + Cl^-)$ (normal range 6–12 mmol/l)

Anion gap = $(143 + 4.5) - (16.2 + 107) = 24.3$

Causes of anion gap metabolic acidosis

Drug poisoning
Lactic acidosis (eg shock, severe hypoxia, acute liver failure)
Renal failure
Ketoacidosis (eg diabetes, starvation)

4.9 D: Commence haemodialysis

Lithium is a drug with limited prescribing indications – its use being almost exclusive to psychiatry. It should only be prescribed on specialist advice. Lithium has a narrow therapeutic window and is dangerous in toxic levels. The desired serum lithium concentration is 0.4–1.2 mmol/l. Patients on lithium require enrolment in a monitoring programme to check that serum levels stay within a narrow desired range.

Indications for prescription of lithium

Treatment and prophylaxis of mania
Prophylaxis of bipolar affective disorder (BAD)
Prophylaxis of recurrent depression
Cluster headaches (unlicensed)

In mild cases of lithium toxicity (>1.2 but <2 mmol/l) discontinuing the drug and giving generous volumes of fluid may suffice. Renal function should be monitored. Diuretics should be avoided. Dehydration or the co-administration of diuretics may be the cause of toxic serum lithium levels.

At toxic levels, especially when renal impairment is present, urgent haemodialysis should be performed.

Key potential side-effects of lithium

Thyroid disease (especially hypothyroidism)
Memory and cognitive impairment
Diabetes insipidus
Renal impairment (renal failure in overdose)

4.10 D: Fibromyalgia

Fibromyalgia is a functional condition of voluntary muscles. It represents a significant burden to both family practice and rheumatology outpatient work. It is an entirely benign condition in which subjective clinical features are at odds to objective findings. The characteristic examination findings are of multiple 'trigger' points over the soft tissues of the neck, intrascapular region and spine. It is most frequent in females in the age range 20–40 years and little if any successful treatments are available. Sufferers typically have a poor sleep pattern which is lacking in the REM component leaving them unrefreshed and almost continuously tired. There is believed to be a large psychogenic element to the condition. Patients are encouraged to establish a regular sleep pattern, sometimes aided by amitriptyline (a tricyclic antidepressant) and to take part in a graded exercise programme. It is important at first presentation to exclude other rheumatological conditions which may initially present in a relatively non-specific manner. All investigations will be normal.

4.11. D: Ischaemic colitis

Ischaemic colitis occurs when the arterial supply to the bowel is compromised. The cause is normally an embolus to either of the mesenteric arteries (superior and inferior) which, if left untreated, may result in unviable ischaemic bowel. A proportion will resolve without surgical intervention. It occurs most commonly at the splenic flexure. This is a 'water-shed' area of arterial supply between the superior and inferior mesenteric arteries. This diagnosis is within the differential for both an acute PR bleed and abdominal pain. A history of atrial fibrillation or clinical manifestations of atherosclerotic disease provide the clue. Diagnosis is either radiologically, ideally with a mesenteric angiogram, or directly at laparotomy. If left untreated perforation and peritonitis can occur. Angiodysplasia is a diagnosis of exclusion.

4.12 C: Pretibial myxoedema

All of the features listed in the stems are clinical features that can be observed in Grave's disease. Grave's disease is one cause of hyperthyroidism. It is an autoimmune disease of the thyroid gland with a significant female preponderance.

However, there are only three features unique to Grave's disease:

- pretibial myxoedema
- thyroid acropachy
- ophthalmoplegia.

4.13 B: To monitor the white cell count

Schizophrenia is treated with anti-psychotic medications which are chiefly divided into typical and atypical agents. Furthermore, maintenance therapy may either be oral or by intramuscular (IM) depot preparations.

The newer atypical agents are said to have a better side-effect profile with particular regard to extra-pyramidal side effects.

Extra-pyramidal side effects

Parkinsonism
Acute dystonia
Akathisia
Tardive dyskinesia

Clozapine is indicated for those patients who fail to respond to two antipsychotics at therapeutic doses, at least one of which should have been an atypical antipsychotic. Although a very effective medication it is not without risks. There is an up to 2% risk of developing agranulocytosis from this medication. Clozapine can cause bone marrow suppression. It is therefore compulsory for all patients on this medication to be enrolled in a monitoring programme with regular blood tests to check the white cell count, being especially intensive on commencement.

Antipsychotic medications

Typical	Atypical
Haloperidol, Chlorpromazine	Olanzapine
Flupenthixol, zuclopenthixol	Risperidone, amisulpride
Trifluoperazine	Quetiapine, Aripiprazole
Sulpiride	Clozapine*

4.14 A: Phenytoin

Phenytoin toxicity presents as a cerebellar syndrome. Phenytoin is one of a small group of commonly prescribed but important medications that have a narrow therapeutic window. These drugs include theophylline, digoxin, lithium and aminoglycoside antibiotics. The line between beneficial treatment effects and deleterious effects to the patient is narrower than with other medications. This requires a minimum of monitoring drug levels on commencement or dose alteration. An alteration is suggested by the recent visit to neurology outpatients. The property responsible for this phenomenon is saturation kinetics. Phenytoin demonstrates a non-linear relationship between dose and plasma concentration. At a certain dose (which will vary between patients) the hepatic metabolising pathway will become 'saturated' so that further drug will give a disproportionately high level in the plasma. A small incremental rise in the oral dose may cause a disproportionately high increase in plasma concentration causing significant side-effects.

4.15 C: Depression with secondary panic attacks

It is important to recognise that panic attacks and other anxiety symptoms can be a secondary feature of other disorders, including depression. It is crucial to consider the temporal development of symptoms. In this case the core symptoms of a depressive episode (low mood, anergia and anhedonia) clearly precede the development of panic attacks. She now expresses some passive suicidal ideation, which should be of concern. The correct diagnosis of depression is important, not least because the appropriate treatment for the panic attacks in this case would be to treat the underlying disorder. As she becomes less depressed her panic attacks should remit.

Panic disorder should be diagnosed where there are recurrent attacks of severe anxiety/panic which are not restricted to any particular situation or set of circumstances, and which are therefore unpredictable. For a definite diagnosis there should be several attacks within a period of a month. It is possible to have isolated panic attacks which do not attract a diagnosis of panic disorder.

Common symptoms of a panic attack

- Sudden onset of palpitations
- Chest pain
- Choking sensations
- Dizziness
- Feelings of unreality (depersonalisation or derealisation)
- Secondary fear of dying, losing control or going mad.

4.16 Deep venous thrombosis   Answers: All false

Deep venous thromboses are common, particularly in immobile patients such as those with fractured neck of femur. Twenty per cent of deep venous thromboses extend proximally and approximately 2% embolise. A duplex ultrasound is the first-line investigation. A venogram should not be performed routinely as it is more invasive and involves a radiation dose to the patient.

The use of low molecular weight heparin injections, which can be given by a district nurse, have made outpatient treatment preferable. Admission is however advised for the following conditions:

- increased risk of bleeding
- bilateral deep venous thromboses
- extension to the inferior vena cava
- pulmonary embolus
- dementia
- intravenous drug abuse.

An above-knee deep venous thrombosis should be treated with 6 months of anticoagulation. Three months of treatment is advised if the thrombus is at the trifurcation, ie where the three main veins of the leg join to form the popliteal vein.

A below-knee deep venous thrombosis may cause clinical problems such as skin changes from venous obstruction. A pulmonary embolus is extremely unlikely and the risks of anticoagulation outweigh the risk of pulmonary embolus.

4.17 Pulmonary embolism   Answers: A D

A pulmonary embolism is unlikely if the arterial oxygen is above 10.7 kPa or if the respiratory rate is <20 respirations per minute. The chest X-ray is often normal in a patient with a pulmonary embolus. D-dimer measurements are useful. If the D-dimer levels are below 0.3 ml/l an acute pulmonary embolus is unlikely. Note that a raised D-dimer is not diagnostic because it is elevated in malignant disease, infection, recent surgery and if the total bilirubin is above 34 ml/l.

Pulmonary embolism occurs in young adults. Those with increased risk are women on the contraceptive pill, patients with a family history of thrombosis, patients who have undergone recent surgery, trauma, immobilisation or those who have a malignancy.

4.18 Asthma   Answers: A C

The features of severe asthma include:

- a peak flow <50% of the patient's best measurement or predicted
- tachycardia >110 bpm irrespective of whether a beta-agonist has been given
- tachypnoea >25 respirations/minute
- unable to complete a whole sentence.

A potentially fatal asthmatic attack is indicated by:

- a peak flow of <33%
- cyanosis/hypoxia
- a silent chest on auscultation – it is important to remember that if no wheeze can be heard this is a bad sign as it implies that air entry into the chest is so poor that a wheeze cannot be generated. Do not interpret the absence of a wheeze to mean that there is no bronchoconstriction
- PCO_2 > 6 kPa suggests fatigue and imminent respiratory failure – the PCO_2 should be low because of hyperventilation
- A previous ITU admission indicates that the patient is prone to life-threatening attacks.

Acute asthma still carries a high mortality. In the UK approximately 2000 people die from this each year. Always remember to have a low threshold for contacting an anaesthetist to ventilate the patient.

4.19 Blood pressure   Answers: A B C D

Patients must be admitted and treated in hospital if the raised blood pressure is causing end-organ damage, eg retinal damage, renal damage, encephalopathy, seizures or coma. Myocardial infarction, dissecting aneurysm and pulmonary oedema may also be caused by a severe rise in blood pressure and are also indications of urgent treatment. Note the blood pressure should be brought down slowly aiming for a diastolic blood pressure of around 110–115 mmHg after 24 h. A sudden drop in blood pressure may precipitate myocardial infarction, stroke and acute renal failure. Intravenous therapy should therefore be avoided and if it is necessary should be given in an ITU setting.

4.20 ECG changes   Answer: D

Diagnostic features of acute myocardial infarction are:

- ST elevation greater than or equal to 1 mm in two adjacent limb leads
- ST elevation of greater than or equal to 2 mm in two adjacent precordial leads
- Left bundle branch block that is new in the context of a convincing history.

Note that if there is a convincing history then any ST elevation may be significant but before thrombolysis the case should be discussed with a senior doctor.

4.21 Contraindications to thrombolysis   Answers: A D

There are major and relative contraindications to thrombolysis. If any of these are present the case should be discussed urgently with a senior doctor, such as the on-call cardiology registrar. The **major contraindications** to thrombolysis are active bleeding or known bleeding disorders and the following specific conditions:

- CNS: previous subarachnoid or intra-cerebral bleed, haemorrhagic stroke, neoplasm aneurysm or AV malformation. A recent stroke within 1 year; head injury or CNS surgery within 6 months.
- Cardiac: suspected aortic dissection. Traumatic cardiopulmonary resuscitation within 1 month.

- GI: acute pancreatitis, oesophageal varices, any recent major surgery or bleeding within 2 months.
- Obstetric: pregnancy; obstetric delivery within 10 days/heavy vaginal bleeding (but not a normal menstruation).
- Orthopaedic: bone fracture within 1 month.

The relative contraindications are:

- CNS: history of stroke with residual deficit, proliferative diabetic retinopathy/laser treatment.
- Cardiac: a blood pressure of >200/110 mmHg; this should be treated first. Puncture of a non-compressible artery within 2 weeks.
- GI: active peptic ulcer disease. Organ biopsy in the last 2 weeks. Tooth extraction within the last month.
- Respiratory: cavitating pulmonary disease.
- Oral anticoagulant therapy is a relative contraindication, as is any minor surgery within the last month.

4.22 Abdominal X-ray   Answers: A C D

Under normal circumstances there is a large amount of gas in the large bowel, a great deal less in the small bowel. The small bowel tends to lie centrally. The ascending and descending colon are normally the most laterally seen loops of bowel. The transverse colon is usually identified crossing the upper abdomen.

In the small bowel the valvulae conniventes are seen as parallel bands, extending fully across the lumen. They are particularly noticeable when the small bowel is distended. Small bowel is abnormally distended if the loops are >3 cm in diameter. The large bowel has haustral folds that extend only one-third across the lumen. The large bowel is dilated if >5.5 cm in diameter.

4.23 Unstable angina   Answer: A

Unstable angina is a term that many cardiologists no longer use. The term was used to describe the clinical syndrome of rapidly worsening, prolonged or increasingly frequent episodes of chest pain, or pain occurring at rest or chest pain of recent onset. Many cardiologists use the term 'acute coronary syndrome' which encompasses the spectrum of conditions with mild ischaemia at one end of the spectrum and myocardial infarction at the other end. The risk of myocardial infarction or death within 6 weeks of developing the above conditions may be as high as 10% and the condition must therefore be taken seriously. The patient must be admitted to hospital and ideally to the Coronary Care Unit. Observation and continuous ECG monitoring should be performed. Intravenous access and blood sample for cardiac troponin levels should also be performed. The treatment involves aspirin, subcutaneous low-molecular-weight heparin, intravenous nitrates and beta-blockade. In patients with unstable angina and high-risk coronary anatomy, there is a case for giving a glycoprotein IIB IIIA receptor antagonist such as abciximab and the case should be discussed with the on-call cardiologist. The cardiologist should also be contacted to discuss patients who fail to improve on the above treatment so that urgent coronary angiography can be considered. Cardiac troponin is highly specific for cardiac damage.

4.24 Gastrointestinal bleed

Answers: A C D E

It is useful to divide patients into high- and low-risk groups to determine management. A patient is high risk if they are hypotensive, there has been a haematemesis or melaena has been passed, tachycardia >100 bpm, postural hypotension and co-morbidity.

The patient is deemed to be low risk if they are <60 years of age, they have had a coffee-ground vomitus and the cardiovascular parameters are stable. Low-risk patients should be admitted and given fluids. They should be observed for signs of further bleeding and an endoscopy should be booked for the next routine list.

Patients at high risk who are unstable, eg with hypotension, require immediate resuscitation and urgent endoscopy in the presence of a surgeon. Patients who are at high risk but who are stable require resuscitation and should have an endoscopy within 12 h.

4.25 Acute asthma

Answers: All false

The treatment of acute asthma is as follows:

- Oxygen: a high concentration of 6 l/min is required as most patients will have a low PCO_2. The issue of low-concentration oxygen is only relevant in CO_2-retaining patients with COPD (chronic obstructive pulmonary disease).
- Bronchodilators: oxygen-driven nebulised bronchodilators such as salbutamol should be started as soon as possible. If there is no improvement these should be repeated at 15-min intervals. Nebulised ipratropium bromide helps in about 30% of patients and can be given every 6 h.
- An IV bronchodilator should only be given if the patient has failed to respond to repeated nebulised treatment.

- Corticosteroids: these should be given as soon as possible as they take 6 h to produce improvement. Intravenous hydrocortisone 200 ml or prednisolone 60 ml orally may be given.
- Magnesium: for patients with severe asthma who respond poorly to nebulised bronchodilators, intravenous magnesium may be given as an infusion. Note the question says oral magnesium and is therefore false.
- Aminophylline: this is rarely given now because of limited efficacy and numerous side-effects.
- Hydration: patients are often dehydrated as they have not been drinking enough because of being unwell and also via extra loss through hyperventilation. Patients should be rehydrated with intravenous fluids.
- Chest X-ray: this should be done to exclude a pneumothorax and to look for supra added infection.

4.26 Jugular venous pressure   Answers: C D

The A wave is due to atrial contraction. The V wave is due to venous return to the right atrium during ventricular systole. Large A waves are due to increased atrial contraction, for example in tricuspid stenosis, pulmonary stenosis and pulmonary hypertension. Tricuspid stenosis causes large A waves but not cannon waves. Cannon waves occur when the right ventricle and atrium contract simultaneously, as in complete heart block or ventricular tachycardia.

The jugular venous pressure (JVP) is raised in congestive cardiac failure but not in pure left ventricular failure.

During inspiration intrathoracic pressure falls, causing blood to be sucked into the right side of the heart. This is responsible for the normal fall in JVP on inspiration. If the right side of the heart is physically prevented from relaxing to accommodate the increase in venous return the venous pressure rises. This occurs in constrictive pericarditis and cardiac tamponade and this paradoxical rise in the JVP is known as Kussmaul's sign.

In tricuspid regurgitation large V waves and a pulsatile liver are features, but the mitral valve is on the LEFT side and therefore has no effect on the JVP.

4.27 Cerebellar lesions   Answers: C D

The features of a cerebellar syndrome may be remembered by the mnemonic **DANISH:**

- **D**ysdiadochokinesis
- **A**taxia (patients have a broad-based gait with a tendency to fall to the side of the lesion; they are unable to walk heel to toe)
- **N**ystagmus
- **I**ntention tremor
- **S**lurred speech
- **H**ypotonia.

The plantar responses are typically flexor and the neurological signs are ipsilateral as the majority of pathways from the cerebellum do not cross over.

4.28 Gastrointestinal malignancy   Answers: A B C D

This is an extremely common question that has been seen in both general medicine and paediatric sections and also in general surgery papers. The stems that have been reported most frequently are C, E and A (in that order).

Familial adenomatous polyposis coli is caused by an autosomal dominant gene on chromosome 5. Multiple polyps occur in the colon during adolescence, and carcinoma typically develops in the third decade. This condition accounts for 1% of all cases of colon cancer.

Recent evidence suggests that *H. pylori* infection increases the risk of gastric lymphoma. Regression of the lymphoma is said to occur on eradication of the infection. Gastric adenocarcinoma is also associated with *H. pylori*.

Coeliac disease causes increased risk of small-bowel lymphoma. When a patient's symptoms persist, despite adhering to a strict gluten-free diet, the development of lymphoma should be strongly suspected. There is also an increased risk of oesophageal carcinoma with coeliac disease.

Peutz-Jeghers syndrome is characterised by buccal pigmentation and small bowel polyps which are non-malignant. Inheritance is autosomal dominant. A few textbooks argue that the polyps have some malignant potential, and there is some evidence of an increase in upper gastrointestinal tract malignancy.

Uncomplicated reflux does not cause malignancy. A condition such as Barrett's oesophagus, which is associated with chronic reflux, does however increase the risk of oesophageal carcinoma.

The risk of oesophageal cancer is also increased in achalasia and in Plummer–Vinson (Patterson–Brown–Kelly) syndrome, the condition of iron deficiency in association with an oesophageal web.

4.29 Benign intracranial hypertension   Answers: A B D E

This condition is more common in obese young women especially if taking drugs such as the oral contraceptive pill, tetracyclines and retinoids. Benign intracranial hypertension (BIH) causes marked papilloedema and can cause blindness. Headaches are a frequent symptom and are caused by the raised intracranial pressure. They improve dramatically post-lumbar puncture, which forms the basis of treatment. The carbonic anhydrase inhibitor acetazolamide is also used. When these methods fail, shunts can be inserted surgically.

4.30 Gynaecomastia   Answers: B C

This is a very common question.

Gynaecomastia refers to enlargement of the male breast due to an increase in breast tissue. Oestrogen is the main hormone responsible for this and hence oestrogen-secreting tumours, such as testicular tumours and certain types of bronchial carcinoma, may cause gynaecomastia. Oestrogen is normally metabolised by the liver and so its levels are increased in liver failure. In chronic renal failure altered hormone binding produces a functional excess of oestrogen.

Human chorionic gonadotropin (hCG) secretion also causes gynaecomastia. Testicular tumours can therefore produce gynaecomastia by production of oestrogen or hCG.

It is a common misconception that prolactin increases breast tissue growth. This is not the case. Hyperprolactinaemia, however, may cause galactorrhoea (ie milk production and secretion) but do not confuse this with gynaecomastia.

Drug causes of gynaecomastia include cimetidine, spironolactone and digoxin.

4.31 Hypoglycaemia   Answers: B C D E

Hypoglycaemia is unusual except in patients with diabetes who are prescribed hypoglycaemic drugs. Occasionally other drugs such as alcohol and aspirin may cause hypoglycaemia. Tumours such as insulinoma and carcinoid also cause hypoglycaemia. Sepsis usually causes hyperglycaemia but may also cause hypoglycaemia especially in neonates.

Glucose must be given IMMEDIATELY. If possible it should be given by mouth but where this is not possible it should be administered intravenously. The oral route is preferable and it is equally effective without the risk of tissue necrosis that may occur with intravenous administration if the needle is not properly sited within a vein.

Diabetic ketoacidosis is the result of a lack of insulin and hyperglycaemia.

4.32 Acute stroke and transient ischaemia   **Answers: B D**

By definition, a transient ischaemic attack resolves within 24 h and often within 1 h. All patients with a stroke should have a CT or MRI scan, preferably within 48 h but more urgently if there is worsening neurology. A scan is needed to differentiate infarction from haemorrhage and exclude other causes of neurology such as tumour, arteriovenous malformation and subarachnoid haemorrhage. The scan will also identify patients requiring urgent surgical referral.

An echocardiogram is only required if there is significant cardiac abnormality on clinical examination or if the patient is <60 years old. Patients who are <50 years old with recurrent unexplained stroke should have a transoesophageal echocardiogram.

An ECG will identify arrhythmia such as atrial fibrillation and should be performed in all patients with a stroke.

Carotid duplex studies are only necessary for a carotid territory stroke or if the territory of the stroke is uncertain.

All patients should have a full blood count, ESR, urea and creatinine and electrolytes, glucose, cholesterol and a chest X-ray. If there is a haemorrhagic stroke (blood is seen on CT/MRI) a clotting screen should be performed. If the patient has had an ischaemic stroke and is below 60 years of age a thrombophilia screen should be performed and autoantibodies and anti-cardiolipin measurements performed.

4.33 Intracranial haemorrhage   **Answers: A C D E**

The term intracranial haemorrhage means that bleeding has occurred within the brain or subarachnoid or subdural or extradural spaces.

Cerebellar haemorrhage is of great concern as there is little space within the posterior fossa and bleeding rapidly causes compression with the danger of herniation and death. Urgent neurosurgical referral is required. A CT scan is very sensitive in detection of blood. However, up to 1% of subarachnoid haemorrhages will have normal CT scan and a lumbar puncture is required to detect the haemorrhage.

A subdural haemorrhage is usually due to a venous bleed. On a CT scan it has a crescentic appearance. An extradural haemorrhage is usually due to an arterial bleed and on a CT scan has a bi-concave or lentiform appearance.

4.34 Status epilepticus
Answers: A C

Status epilepticus is defined as either continuous, generalised, tonic-clonic seizures or tonic-clonic seizures that are so frequent that each attack begins before the post-ictal period of the preceding one ends.

The mortality is high and it is important to control the fits as soon as possible. As with all medical emergencies management begins with ABC, ie airway, breathing and circulation.

Make the environment safe for the patients, eg using padded bed rails to keep the patient from being damaged. When possible, place the patient in a semi-prone position with the head down, maintain airway and help prevent aspiration. If possible, during an inter-ictal period, insert an airway and administer oxygen.

Set up an intravenous line as soon as possible and send venous blood for measurement of glucose, urea and electrolytes, calcium, liver function, full blood count and clotting, and anticonvulsant blood levels.

The blood glucose should be assessed rapidly using a BM test and if the patient is hypoglycaemic 50% glucose should be administered rapidly, but do not wait for the formal blood glucose level to come back from the laboratory.

Check body temperature and blood pressure and do an ECG.

If possible get a history from an accompanying person and look for clues on the patient that might help with management such as a medic alert bracelet. The seizures should be terminated with a benzodiazepine such as lorazepam or diazepam. The patient should also be given IV phenytoin which will help stop seizures if they are still continuing and also prevent further ones.

If seizures do not stop on this regime, the patient should be transferred to an ITU and a neurological opinion urgently sought.

4.35 Charcoal
Answers: C D E

Activated charcoal both decreases absorption of most drugs and increases elimination by interrupting the entero-enteric and entero-hepatic circuits. It will not work with mineral acids, lithium, DDT, cyanide or ferrous sulphate.

It is by far the most effective treatment for most drugs and should be considered the treatment of choice in the first 1.5 h after overdose, with or without gastric lavage preceding the dose. Some drugs such as tricyclic and opiates delay gastric emptying and so lavage and activated charcoal can be performed even if overdosage was up to 12 h earlier.

4.36 Resting tremor

Answers: A B D

The cerebellar tremor is an intention tremor and does not typically occur at rest. Causes of a resting tremor include anxiety, beta-agonist drugs, alcohol intoxication or withdrawal, thyrotoxicosis, familial tremor and basal ganglia lesions, for example, Parkinson's disease. Note that the tremor of Parkinson's is a pill rolling rest tremor which decreases on intentional movement in contrast to a cerebellar tremor.

4.37 Coagulation

Answers: B C

The extrinsic and intrinsic pathways lead to the final common pathway; this results in thrombin production which activates fibrinogen conversion to fibrin, allowing clot formation. The extrinsic pathway involves tissue thromboplastin and factor VII and is measured by the prothrombin time (PT time). The intrinsic pathway involves XII, XI, IX, VIII, platelet phospholipid and calcium. The final common pathway involves factors X, V, calcium and formation of II (prothrombin). The intrinsic pathway and final common pathway are measured by the APTT (also known as the PTT and the KCCT). The conversion of fibrinogen to fibrin by thrombin is measured by the thrombin time (TT). Temporal arteritis is a vasculitis and does not affect the clotting pathway.

4.38 Randomised controlled clinical trials

Answer: D

A double-blind randomised controlled trial is the ideal way of assessing efficacy of a drug. The term double-blind means that neither the patient nor the doctor knows whether the patient is receiving the drug or a placebo, or the drug being studied and an established drug for comparison. The study may be done in parallel or cross-over. In the latter one group of patients starts on the new drug and are then swapped over to the old drug or placebo. The other group is started on the established treatment or placebo and then changed over to the drug being studied.

The more patients that are studied the better, so that the less common side-effects can be picked up.

4.39 Complications of IV drug abuse

Answers: A B C D

Apart from the side-effects of the drugs involved, IV drug abuse has numerous problems. Needle sharing transmits blood-borne viruses such as HIV, hepatitis B and hepatitis C. Hepatitis A is water borne and transmitted by the faeco-oral route.

An infected needle allows bacteria to reach the heart, in particular the valves, producing endocarditis. It is theoretically possible for microorganisms to reach the brain, causing a cerebral abscess but a right to left shunt would be required for this. Dirty needles may also allow tetanus to be introduced. Large particles injected into a vein, particularly the large femoral vein, could produce a significant pulmonary embolus.

4.40 Sickle cell anaemia associations   Answers: A B D

Sickle cell anaemia does not present at birth, as fetal haemoglobin is still present. When cells sickle they block small vessels causing infarction and damage to numerous organs. For example, splenic infarction results in a small spleen. In the kidneys tubular dysfunction occurs causing a defective urinary concentrating ability. Bone infarction causes pain (painful dactylitis in toddlers) and also increases the risk of osteomyelitis. Patients who have a reduced splenic function are also at risk of overwhelming septicaemia from *Pneumococcus* and *Meningococcus* in particular. A chest crisis may occur: severe shunting and hypoxia caused by intrapulmonary sickling may spread throughout the lungs, mimicking pulmonary embolism and pneumonia. Cerebral sickling causes the patient to have fits, strokes, coma, bizarre behaviour or psychosis.

If sickling occurs within the splanchnic bed the patient may develop abdominal pain with signs of peritonism and jaundice, which is known as girdle syndrome.

4.41 Mitral stenosis   Answers: B E

The presence of a third heart sound, a displaced apex beat and an early diastolic murmur make the diagnosis of mitral stenosis unlikely.

Symptoms of mitral stenosis:

- Dyspnoea – as the left atrium hypertrophies the left atrial pressure rises. The pulmonary venous pressure then rises causing pulmonary venous hypertension. Increased venous pressure in any part of the body will produce oedema and in the lungs it is referred to as pulmonary oedema.
- Fatigue, weakness – the low cardiac output which occurs with valve stenoses gives rise to this. Development of cor pulmonale exacerbates these symptoms.
- Palpitations – atrial fibrillation occurs secondary to the enlarged left atrium.
- Emboli – atrial fibrillation increases the risk of thrombosis and pulmonary and systemic emboli.

- Dysphagia – rarely, the enlarged left atrium compresses the oesophagus to produce dysphagia.

Signs of mitral stenosis:

- Inspection – mitral facies.
- Pulse – this is irregular in both rate and volume – this is the correct way to describe the pulse in atrial fibrillation.
- Precordium
  - o Palpation – right ventricular heave, tapping apex beat – not displaced because the ventricle is normal in size.
  - o Auscultation – the first heart sound is loud (the stenosed valve slams shut). A loud P2 occurs with pulmonary hypertension and an opening snap may be heard as the valve opens in diastole. If the left atrial pressure is very high, as with severe mitral stenosis, the valve may open earlier. Therefore the opening snap is heard earlier, ie closer to the second heart sound.

There is a mid-diastolic, low-pitched rumbling murmur best heard with the bell, just lateral to the apex beat. It is best heard in the left lateral position in expiration and is increased with exercise. Pre-systolic accentuation may occur if the patient is in sinus rhythm as atrial contraction forces more blood through the valve, increasing the turbulence and hence the loudness of the murmur.

4.42 Intercostal chest drain   Answers: All false

A narrow bore intercostal chest drain is used for draining a pneumothorax and should be inserted pointing upwards. Drainage for an effusion is with a large bore drain and is inserted pointing downwards.

Insertion should be by blunt dissection; a trocar is no longer recommended. For greatest safety the chest drain should be inserted in the triangle bounded by the apex of the axilla, the nipple (4th intercostal space in the mid-clavicular line) and the base of the scapula.

4.43 Haemoptysis   Answers: A B D E

Haemoptysis refers to the coughing up of blood or blood-stained sputum. This will occur if there is damage to the bronchi or air spaces, or damage to the blood vessels. It is less likely to occur when damage is of the interstitial lung tissues, for example lung fibrosis.

Diseases of the bronchi and its connections:

- Primary tumours – secondary tumours tend to metastasise to the interstitium

- Infection – pneumonia, lung abscess, TB
- Bronchial wall damage – for example, cystic fibrosis, bronchiectasis.

Lesions of the blood vessel:

- Lumen – for example, pulmonary embolus
- Wall – vasculitis, for example Goodpasture's, Wegener's and Churg–Strauss syndromes.

Raised pulmonary venous pressure, for example mitral stenosis, and left ventricular failure make the vessels more liable to rupture and bleed.

4.44 Renal biopsy   Answers: A B C D

Consent is required for all invasive procedures. If a patient will not consent or is uncooperative, no invasive procedure should be performed.

Most renal biopsies are performed to determine the underlying cause of renal failure. If the kidneys are small and shrunken this implies the disease process has already gone too far and determining a diagnosis at this stage is too late. Also, small kidneys are difficult to biopsy and histology is difficult to interpret.

A biopsy may be taken from a single post-transplant kidney when rejection appears to be occurring. However, if a non-transplant patient has only one kidney, this should not be biopsied as 1 in 400 patients have profuse post-biopsy haemorrhage requiring occlusion of the bleeding vessel at angiography or even nephrectomy.

Repeated renal biopsies are often necessary to determine rejection or to monitor response to treatment.

4.45 Skin conditions associated with malignancy   Answers: A B E

Dermatomyositis occurs with increased incidence in carcinoma of the bronchus and ovaries. A purplish discoloration around the eyelids and knuckles is characteristic.

Acanthosis nigricans is a dark velvety rash especially under the axilla. It is associated with gastric and other intra-abdominal malignancy. Ninety per cent of patients with acanthosis nigricans have a malignancy.

Mycosis fungoides is a T-cell lymphoma initially confined to the skin. Erythema gyratum repens consists of concentric erythematous rings over the whole body. It is associated with carcinoma of the bronchus.

Necrolytic migratory erythema is associated with glucagonoma.

Migrating thrombophlebitis is associated with carcinoma of the pancreas. Ichthyosis is skin thickening associated with lymphoma.

Eczema and psoriasis are not associated with malignancy. Psoriasis can be treated with methotrexate which increases the risk of haemopoietic malignancy, but the question refers to the skin condition and not to the treatment.

4.46 Diabetic patients   Answers: A D

Drivers treated with insulin or oral diabetic drugs are required to notify the DVLA of their condition. Drivers of heavy goods vehicles or public service vehicles whose diabetes is controlled by diet alone must also notify the DVLA.

Insulin may be extracted from pork or beef pancreas but beef insulins are rarely used. Human sequence insulin may be produced by enzymatic modification of porcine insulin or synthetically by DNA technology. All insulin preparations are immunogenic in humans but this rarely causes a problem in clinical practice. It was thought that human insulin would have many advantages over porcine insulin but this has not been established in clinical trials. In fact, some patients have found that switching to human insulin after having had porcine insulin has caused a reduction in the warning symptoms of hypoglycaemia and these patients have been put back on porcine insulin.

Insulin is inactivated by gastrointestinal enzymes and cannot be given orally. It must be given by injection.

During illness stress hormones such as cortisol cause blood glucose levels to rise. During an illness a diabetic patient is particularly at risk of hyperglycaemia even if they are not eating, and insulin is absolutely necessary. In fact higher doses may be needed.

Diabetic patients taking metformin are at increased risk of lactic acidosis when radiological intravenous contrast agents are given. Most radiology departments recommend that metformin is stopped for 48 h after performing a procedure such as intravenous urogram and renal function should be checked before restarting the metformin.

4.47 High-dose oxygen   Answers: A B D E

In conditions where hypoventilation is likely, such as chronic obstructive pulmonary disease, high-dose oxygen must not be given. Hypoventilation produces a rise in CO_2 and a fall in PO_2; in time the respiratory centres within the brain are reset to tolerate a chronically high PCO_2 and so these patients then rely on their low PO_2 to produce a hypoxic drive for ventilation; if high-concentration oxygen is given this drive is abolished and the patient may stop breathing altogether.

High-dose oxygen (ie up to a concentration of 60%) is appropriate when conditions produce hyperventilation such as an acute asthmatic attack, pneumonia, pulmonary embolism and fibrosing alveolitis. In these conditions a low partial pressure of oxygen is associated with a normal or low PCO_2.

An important exception is a life-threatening attack of asthma. The patient may become so exhausted that hypoventilation results, causing a decrease in arterial oxygen tension and a rise in PCO_2. In this case a high concentration of oxygen is required despite the hypoventilation (this is an acute situation and the patient does not normally rely on a hypoxic drive) and positive pressure ventilation should be urgently considered.

4.48 Lipid-lowering drugs   Answers: C D E

Lowering the concentration of low-density lipoprotein (LDL) cholesterol and raising high-density (HDL) cholesterol reduces the progression of coronary atherosclerosis and may even induce regression.

There is evidence that if LDL cholesterol can be lowered by 25–35%, primary and secondary prevention of coronary heart disease is achieved. Treatment with statins has been shown to reduce myocardial infarction, coronary deaths and overall mortality.

Statins are drugs of first choice for treating hypercholesterolaemia and fibrates for treating hypertriglyceridaemia. Statins and fibrates can also be used either together or alone to treat mixed hyperlipidaemia.

4.49 Primary tumours   Answers: A C D

There are four important tumours which commonly metastasise to the lungs. These are carcinoma of the breast, carcinoma of the bronchus, thyroid cancer and renal cancer. Note that this is the same list as metastasise to the bone, with the exception of prostate cancer which does not commonly metastasise to the lung but commonly metastasises to bone.

4.50 Colitis   Answers: B D E

Infective causes of colitis include amoebiasis, *Shigella*, *Salmonella*, *Yersinia*, *Campylobacter*, *E. coli* O157 and *Clostridium difficile* (pseudomembranous colitis).

In immunocompromised hosts other infections such as cytomegalovirus and herpes should also be considered.

Tapeworm infection causes anaemia and weight loss. Influenza is a respiratory tract infection and does not affect the colon.

Other causes of colitis include inflammatory bowel disease, radiation, ischaemic colitis and drugs such as gold.

4.51 Audit studies   Answers: C D

All doctors are now expected to perform audit studies. Audit will also form part of an annual appraisal of each senior hospital doctor as part of clinical governance, which is the legal responsibility of all Trusts. Appraisal will also be necessary for revalidation – that is the process where each doctor will submit a profile of their performance to the GMC in order to stay on the Medical Register. This revalidation process will be done every 5 years.

Audit is therefore extremely important to each doctor (and medical students who are also being asked to perform audit studies).

Audit involves the following:

- a standard should be selected, eg all discharge summaries should be done within 2 days of the patient's discharge from hospital
- assess the local practice, eg patients discharged last week
- compare with the target
- implement change
- re-audit to assess whether improvement has occurred.

Audit is not research and there are many important differences. Research is more precise, involves larger sample sizes and a longer timescale and has strictly defined methodology. Research compares different things whereas audit is comparing the same activities. Research is experimental whereas audit is observational, making it very susceptible to bias. A good audit study should have a standard error and confidence intervals.

4.52 Autonomic neuropathy   Answers: A B C D

One of the complications of diabetes mellitus is an autonomic neuropathy. The features of this include postural hypotension, loss of sinus arrhythmia (pulse does not slow in response to the Valsalva manoeuvre), loss of sweating, impotence, nocturnal diarrhoea, urine retention and incontinence.

4.53 Horner's syndrome
Answers: B C D E

Horner's syndrome consists of ptosis and a constricted pupil (meiosis). Enophthalmos (the eye appears sunken) and anhidrosis (absence of sweating) may also be present. The sympathetic nervous system has a complicated pathway, and damage at various sites will result in a Horner's syndrome. For example, carcinoma of the lung apex may damage the T1 sympathetic ganglion. A thyroid malignancy or trauma to the neck will damage the sympathetic fibres here. A carotid arterial lesion such as a carotid aneurysm or dissection or peri-carotid tumour would have a similar effect. Brainstem lesions such as a stroke, syringobulbia and tumour can also result in a Horner's syndrome. Syringomyelia is a rare lesion affecting the upper cervical chord and may cause a bilateral Horner's syndrome.

Herpes zoster infection of the geniculate ganglion results in a facial nerve palsy and not Horner's syndrome.

4.54 Myasthenia gravis
Answers: C D

Tests for myasthenia gravis include:

- Tensilon test – edrophonium is given intravenously and if muscle strength improves dramatically myasthenia gravis is likely.
- acetylcholine receptor antibodies – these occur in up to 90% of cases and false-positive results are rare. Anti-striated muscle antibody is detectable in 90% of patients with thymoma but is not a specific test.
- electromyogram – in myasthenia gravis repetitive stimulation at low frequency causes a progressive reduction in muscle action potential amplitudes if that particular muscle is affected.
- investigation for the presence of a thymoma include a chest X-ray and thoracic CT scan.

4.55 Cataract
Answers: A B C D

The likelihood of developing a cataract increases with age. Causes include diabetes mellitus and Cushing's syndrome. Steroids will also increase the risk of cataract formation. Ocular disease such as glaucoma, irradiation and trauma to the eye are also causes. Hereditary or congenital cataracts occur in conditions such as dystrophia myotonica.

4.56 Electrocardiogram
Answer: C

Although it is known as the 12-lead ECG this refers to 12 vectors. Only 10 electrodes are actually used to obtain these so-called 12 leads. V1 selects activity in the right ventricle, V3–V4 in the interventricular septum and

V5–V6 in the left ventricle; 2, 3 and AVF record from the inferior surface and 1, AVL and V6 face the lateral wall of the left ventricle. The normal axis is –30 to +90. Less than –30 would indicate left axis deviation and greater than +90 indicates right axis deviation.

Up-sloping depression is a non-specific finding; down-sloping or planar ST depression >1 mm indicates myocardial ischaemia.

The PR interval is recorded from the start of the P wave to the start of the QRS complex. The ST segment is the period between the end of the QRS complex and the start of the T wave.

4.57 Parietal lobe lesion   Answers: C D E

Primitive reflexes, such as the grasp reflex and rooting reflex, are signs of a frontal lobe lesion. Other signs of frontal lobe lesion include emotional lability, intellectual impairment, personality change, urinary incontinence and mono- or hemiparesis. Damage to the left frontal region produces Broca's aphasia.

Parietal lobe lesions produce a variety of signs. Damage to either parietal lobe will produce contralateral sensory loss or neglect (another term is sensory hemi-inattention). Constructional apraxia, agraphaesthesia, a failure to recognise surroundings, limb apraxia and homonymous field defect are also signs. The homonymous defect affecting the parietal lobe alone will produce a homonymous quadrantanopia affecting the lower quadrant compared with an upper field defect which occurs with a temporal lobe lesion.

Specific damage to the right parietal region causes a dressing apraxia, and a failure to recognise faces, as well as the above. Damage to the left parietal region can produce Gerstmann's syndrome, consisting of dyscalculia, dysgraphia and left to right disorientation. Although it is not scientific and should not be quoted in an exam, it is helpful to think of the parietal lobes as being responsible for position in space and in addition to this the right lobe is also concerned with the artistic sociable side, whereas the left is the more studious and mathematical side.

4.58 Pulmonary fibrosis
Answers: A B C D

There are many causes of pulmonary fibrosis and it is helpful to think of causes of upper zone fibrosis separately from mid/lower zone fibrosis.

Causes of upper zone fibrosis can be remembered by the mnemonic

BREAST:
Berylliosis
Radiation
Extrinsic allergic alveolitis
Ankylosing spondylitis
Sarcoid
TB

Of all of these, the most important at undergraduate level are TB and sarcoidosis.

Lower zone shadowing is caused by the connective tissue diseases, for example lupus, rheumatoid arthritis, scleroderma; drugs such as cytotoxics, amiodarone, nitrofurantoin; and the occupational lung diseases, for example silicosis, asbestosis.

Pulmonary fibrosis is not caused by emphysema, chronic bronchitis or asthma.

4.59 Multiple myeloma
Answers: A B C D

Multiple myeloma is due to a monoclonal neoplastic proliferation of plasma cells. These produce abnormal paraprotein which causes hypergammaglobulinaemia (because the total immunoglobulin is measured). However, the abnormal globulin suppresses the useful globulin resulting in immune paresis and hence susceptibility to infection. The paraprotein is usually IgG. It may spill over into the urine causing Bence–Jones proteinuria. The bone marrow is unable to function properly and anaemia, neutropenia and thrombocytopenia occur commonly. The malignant plasma cells in the marrow also cause bone destruction resulting in pathological fractures, hypercalcaemia and raised alkaline phosphatase.

The diagnosis is made by:

- full blood count – looking for the above
- serum electrophoresis – this will show the abnormal paraprotein
- ESR – this is considerably raised
- U&Es, creatinine – renal failure is caused by paraprotein deposition in the renal tubules

- alkaline phosphatase and calcium – because of bone damage
- urine – Bence–Jones protein
- skeletal survey – multiple lytic lesions may be apparent, particularly in the skull, pelvis and long bones
- bone marrow biopsy – >10% of the plasma cells in the marrow are malignant.

Serum electrophoresis, skeletal survey and bone marrow biopsy are the most significant investigations for diagnosis.

4.60 Raynaud's phenomenon   Answers: A B D

Raynaud's phenomenon consists of spasm of the arteries supplying the fingers and toes causing a characteristic colour change, the order of which can be remembered by the mnemonic **WBC** (white blood cell):

White
Blue
Crimson (red)

Raynaud's phenomenon is a common disease affecting 5% of the population, occurring predominantly in young women. It is usually bilateral and the fingers are affected more commonly than the toes. It is precipitated by cold and relieved by warmth. Causes include connective tissue disorders, particularly systemic sclerosis, cryoglobulinaemia, side-effect of beta-blocking drugs, presence of a cervical rib and working with vibrating tools. If there is no underlying cause, the term Raynaud's disease is used rather than Raynaud's phenomenon.

Treatment:

- Treatment of the underlying disease
- Stop smoking
- Precipitating drugs should be avoided and the hands and feet should be kept warm; electrically heated gloves and socks may help; nifedipine, a vasodilator, may also be used.

Diabetes mellitus affects both the large and small blood vessels, but does not specifically produce Raynaud's phenomenon.

Buerger's disease is a condition found in young men who smoke, causing inflammation of the small vessels of the lower limbs. It may be severe enough to require amputation.

_____ END _____

INDEX

The numbers after each entry refer to the paper and question number.

Index